"**Barbara J. Semple** has assembled one of the best collections of self-healing tips anywhere. She is a master in this field, a true inspiration."

–**Richard L. Shames**, *M.D., practicing physician, author of* Thyroid Power *and* Feeling Fat, Fuzzy or Frazzled

[Healing Touch Quick Steps] are "Great healing consciousness and wisdom, presented very well with clarity, and really easy to understand. The **Complete Breath Hug** feels deeply nurturing."

–**Nathan Sivananda**, *D.C., Holistic Chiropractor*

"For nearly 25 years I have witnessed Barbara's tremendous journey of self-healing and am grateful that the Planet has such an enlightened healer and teacher. The *Personal Power Cards* were one of the first tools that Barbara shared. They work just as well today in assisting me to unblock old patterns of thinking and living."

–**Anna Parkins**, *Owner, Sound Energy Plus*

"I had th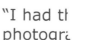 photogr... her new book. It had been over 10 years since I had shot her last, and the transformation was incredible! In total honesty, Barbara looked 10 years younger than the last time we had been together 10 years earlier! This woman walks her talk."

–**Lani Phillips**, *Rare Images Photography and Wisdom of the Crone Cards*

"The Quick Steps help me transmute unpleasant feelings into feelings of peace, tranquility and relaxation, while bathing my body in calmness and self love. I know they are helping on very deep levels."

–**Jill Crosby**, *Owner/Founder www. SpiritualSingles.com*

"I recommend every stressed-out exec, entrepreneur, businessperson, basically everybody, get a copy of *Healing Touch Quick Steps Home Guide*. Move over, Deepak Chopra!"

–**Stefanie Hartman**, *CEO, SHE Inc. and Founder MIT Program and Private JV Club*

INSTANT HEALING

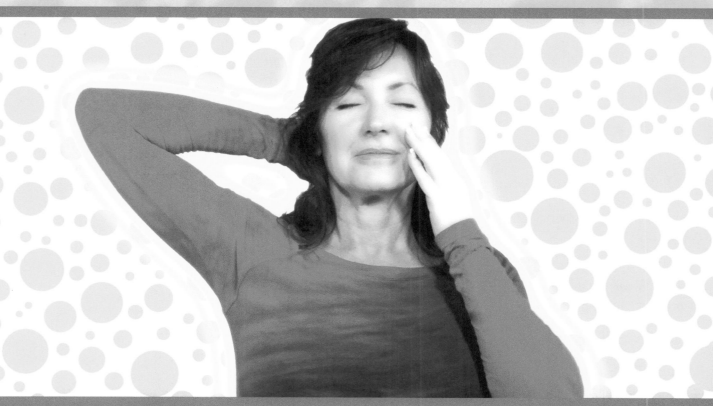

Accessing Creative Intelligence for Healing Body and Soul

Barbara J. Semple

Copyrights and Disclaimers

Copyright@stsci.edu from hubblesite.org with credit to: NASA, H. Ford (JHU), G. Illingworth (UCSC/LO), M.Clampin (STScI), G. Hartig (STScI), the ACS Science Team, and ESA. The ACS Science Team: H. Ford, G. Illingworth, M. Clampin, G. Hartig, T. Allen, K. Anderson, F. Bartko, N. Benitez, J. Blakeslee, R. Bouwens, T. Broadhurst, R. Brown, C. Burrows, D. Campbell, E. Cheng, N. Cross, P. Feldman, M. Franx, D. Golimowski, C. Gronwall, R. Kimble, J. Krist, M. Lesser, D. Magee, A. Martel, W. J. McCann, G. Meurer, G. Miley, M. Postman, P. Rosati, M. Sirianni, W. Sparks, P. Sullivan, H. Tran, Z. Tsvetanov, R. White, and R. Woodruff.

Book cover design, interior pages layout design, and model photography by Nikolas Allen.
www.nikolasallen.com
Nature photography and layout edit by Tom Semple.
Author photography by Lani Phillips.
www.wisdomofthecrone.com.
Original artwork of hand with colored fingers by Lynne Pflueger, Jin Shin Jyutsu teacher and practitioner.
Humpback whales photo on Page 3 by Lisa Denning, www.OceanEyesPhotography.com

Healing Touch Quick Steps
Compassionate Healing Instruction LLC
PO Box 480
Mt. Shasta, CA 96067

To order additional books as well as the multi-media Healing Touch Quick Steps HOME GUIDE, please visit our website: www.healingtouchquicksteps.com

You may also enjoy visiting www.BeTheHarmony.com for articles and tips by the author.

Dedication

In loving memory of my teachers
Mary Ino Burmeister and **Jiro Murai**,
whose perseverance, passion, and commitment
to Knowing Thyself continue to be examples for me.
Thank you thank you thank you.

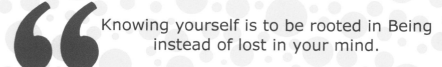

Knowing yourself is to be rooted in Being
instead of lost in your mind.

–Eckhart Tolle

"The skin is the royal robe of mankind where the microcosm and the macrocosm meet."

–Paracelsus

"The universe expands, creates new elements, gives birth to stars and galaxies that start young and grow old, changing in appearance and activity."

–Science News, *February 14, 2009*

"Go beyond the field of thought, the field of emotions, the field of ego, the field of personality, and there's only one field left. That's who we are: the field of pure consciousness localizing as a person."

–Deepak Chopra, *MD*

"What makes the heart beat? What makes breathing possible? What makes digestion possible? What makes the car engine start when you turn on the key? What makes the car lights turn on? The answer to the last two questions would simply be: The BATTERY of the car. The battery is the necessary energy source for the various functions of the car. The answer to what is energy for the body would simply be: The BATTERY of Life. Energy source is necessary for the various functions of the body."

–Mary Burmeister

"We are the container within which all things exist, the bridge between the creations of our inner and outer worlds...regardless of what we call it or how science and religion define it...a force, a field, a presence...links us with one another, our world and a greater power."

–Gregg Braden, *The Divine Matrix*

A huge thank you goes to all of my students and clients over the years for your enthusiasm of this magnificent healing art, for doing your own self-help, and for sharing your "Quick Steps in Action" stories.

Thank you to Stefanie and Tania Hartman for urging me onto the path of creating *Healing Touch Quick Steps* by asking me what I love to do and how can I do it better.

Thank you, Drs. Richard and Karilee Shames, for being my holistic health allies all these years. Monks at Shasta Abbey, thank you for your encouragement.

Very special Thank Yous to: Staycee Margart, our model, for going the distance with long hours of photo shoots and poses. You are lovely. To Dee Sponsler, namaste. To Nikolas Allen, your ideas really transformed this book. You are an amazing artiste. To Jessie Zapffe, for your careful proofreading and your friendship. To Nancy Javor, Rosemary D. and Jill Crosby, Beloved Cheerleaders! Thank you, Lisa Denning, for the awesome humpback whale picture, and Lily Stephen for the Lama Govinda quote.

Thanks to everyone at Xlibris for your help in birthing this beautiful book.

Thank you to David Burmeister for your friendship and encouragement. And thank you to Lynne Pflueger, Anita Willoughby, Janet Oliver, Muriel Carlton, and Jill Holden - five most extraordinary women.

Continuous waves of thanks go to you, Tom. I have loved your creative genius from the day we met. You have an exquisite eye for photographing Nature.

I also thank all of the pioneers of the frontier science now bridging spirituality and science, including Edgar Cayce, Deepak Chopra, M.D., Lynne McTaggart, especially your report of findings about Earth's energies and the Field; Mary Burmeister, Dr. Joan Boryshenko, Dr. Christiane Northrup, Dr. Bruce Lipton, Maureen Redl, MFCC, Susan Weed, ND; Dr. Clarissa Pinkola-Estes, Jean Houston, Dr. Richard Shames, Dr. Karilee Shames, Peggy McColl, Jill Bolte Taylor, Dr. Gladys McGarey, Julie Motz, Dr. Larry Dossey, Gary Zukav, Gregg Braden, Gary DeRodriquez, Eckhart Tolle, Dr. Mehmet Oz, and Oprah Winfrey, among many others. I so appreciate your compassion and dedication to being the change and possibilities you see for humanity.

And thank you, Reader. It is for you that I created this so that you may feel nourished, nurtured, uplifted and supported to thrive as your very best Self. Have fun knowing and being the harmony in your life. Many blessings!

Contents

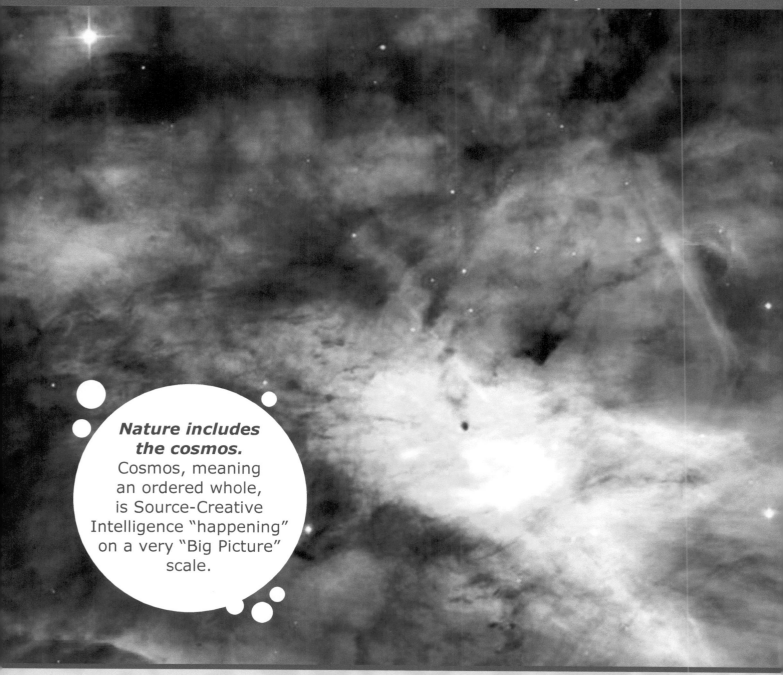

Nature includes the cosmos.
Cosmos, meaning an ordered whole, is Source-Creative Intelligence "happening" on a very "Big Picture" scale.

Source-Creative Intelligence shows us in all things Its magnitude and magnificence to renew, recharge and sustain us.

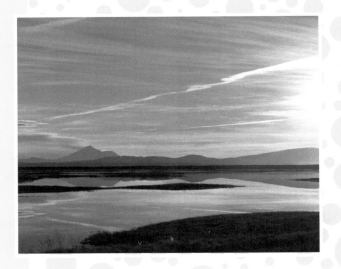

Nature and healing are directly linked to Source.

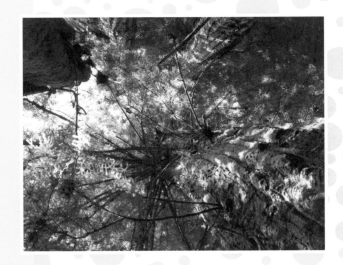

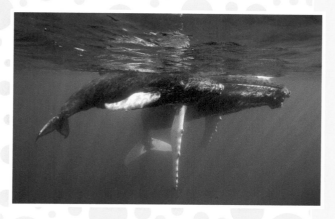

A universal, infinite life force pulses through everything.

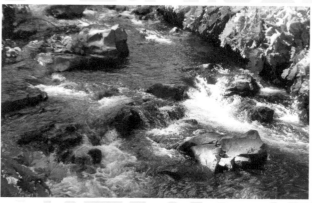

Ever-flowing, infinitely loving and infinitely truthful,

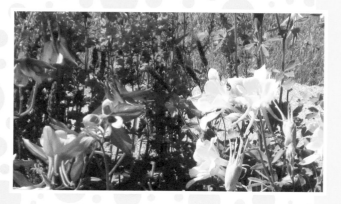

Animating, nourishing and supporting us in every cell in every moment.

From a very early age I always wanted to have a personal relationship with God. As a young Catholic schoolgirl singing Latin at daily masses, I felt very close to God. As I grew older and experienced the natural self-individuation all humans do, my yearning for a deeper knowing of God who not only listened but actually responded and interacted with me, continued to be my "raison d'etre" (reason for being).

When I found the healing art of *Jin Shin Jyutsu*®, I knew my reason for being had finally found profound support with many other people also enthusiastic about being in relationship intimately with God.

The energy healing self-help of *Healing Touch Quick Steps* is primarily based on *Jin Shin Jyutsu* and is a universal art.

This book is a thesis on bridging science and spirituality with quotes and information from various experts including Mary Burmeister that makes a "case" so to speak for the reality, not just a possibility, of every person knowing and engaging a beautiful, active "cause and effect," ask and "receive and give back" relationship with Source.

Through pictures, quotes from leading scientists, mystics and holy women and men, as well as energy healing self-help, you now have access to Creative Intelligence for healing body and soul.

In the Beginning...
What if there was nothing you had to do in life except to allow yourself to be loved? You don't have to go to work or make a living. Every need you have is taken care of before you even know you need it.

What if there was nothing you had to do except be receptive to love? What would you do? Would you do anything? Would you feel bored? Would you feel overflowing with love and contentment and want to share it with others? Would you want to help others who didn't feel as loved as you? Would you want to create from this environment of all there is is love? How would you do things differently?

What if there was nothing you had to do in life except receive love? Would you know how? Would you want to stay in this place of knowing, being and receiving unconditional love all the time, forever?

Preface

Instant healing is an idea whose time has come. It is a growing wave of understanding that suggests you and Source of All Life are One, and, you co-create your life together.

Nearly 25 years ago a teacher told me that humans, each one of us, are a directly linked representative of an ever-evolving, ever-expanding consciousness of the Creator. That one suggestion became a guiding force for the rest of my life's spiritual journey.

Some years later I found the healing art of *Jin Shin Jyutsu*®, from which I would learn that Creator-Creatrix-Source was ever flowing through me and that I could connect with it for my physical healing. And besides that, this idea was true, Infinite Truth (IT), for everyone.

Here was the same message from two very different persons saying the same thing: that you and I are a directly linked part of Creative Intelligence.

Instant Healing – Accessing Creative Intelligence for Healing Body and Soul is mainly a picture book showing you how to apply *Healing Touch Quick Steps* with an emphasis on powerful things you can do instantly to bring your body into harmony that just happen to be opportunities for you to have your own personal relationship with Source while improving your health and well being.

From a place of tender stillness and compassion, you begin to listen with your fingertips and feel Source energy pulsing and responding to your requests.

Does instant healing mean "instant curing"? Not in this book. The first definition I find in the dictionary for the verb *"to heal"* is this: *"to make healthy, whole, or sound; restore to health; free from ailment."* On one level, you are already whole, healthy, and free from ailment. There are many names for this level: the Absolute, the Cosmic, God, the Divine Spirit, Eternal Spirit, Source of All Sources, Creator, Creatrix, Creative Intelligence, or Pure Consciousness.

This is the One Constant and it is the universal manifestation of this One Constant, the spiritual essence that pervades all things. Source is bigger and more powerful than any possible earthly disturbance – bigger than plutonium, bigger than global warming – yes, bigger and more powerful than any possible earthly disturbance. Source is the One Constant power we can count on and we can personally connect with through our bodies. This is important because Source, Eternal Spirit, Stillness, or Silence – spelled with a capital "S" - is the level that you engage as you are actively participating in your life's wholeness with *Healing Touch Quick Steps*.

There are ways to align your body and soul, your earthly life, with your true nature of wholeness, and *Healing Touch Quick Steps* is one of those ways. With the Quick Steps in this book, you may begin to recognize the magnificence of your body and its capacity not only to connect you to what is most Sacred; also to ask and receive help from the Divine with "access codes."

A fine ribbon of ancient wisdom is woven throughout this book so that you may try out a personal relationship with Source, Creative Intelligence. To feel IT pulsing through you as a palpable and interactive force is an awesome thing.

When you do a self-help daily practice as little as 5 minutes a day, your options for instantly helping yourself become second nature. It is like exercising – the more you do it, the more fit you become. In this case, the more energy "fit" you are. The goodness builds on itself – the more you love yourself, the more you care for yourself. Then from that state of being joy and feeling loved and content, Infinite Truth can access you! You and the present moment become One. Ah.

Logically, please
Being responsible for what you create is the first step of self-healing. When you put your hands or fingertips on your body with *Healing Touch Quick Steps*, at places where tensions typically gather, you are able to relieve tension and stress, the relief of which results in all kinds of wonderful benefits like:

- *Increasing circulation*
- *Improving digestion and elimination*
- *Boosting your immune system*
- *Balancing your emotions*
- *Encouraging weight balance*
- *Toning your skin for a natural face lift*
- *Relaxing to sleep*
- *Reviving mental clarity*
- *Engaging a "fountain of youth"*
- *Adding spice to your love life*

Your body needs energy to heal. Without enough vitality it is like asking your car to run on an empty gas tank. You may begin by seeking relief and soon, as you apply these *Healing Touch Quick Steps*, you become aware of your body-mind-spirit strengths. *Instant Healing* is not about focusing on your problems. It is about building on your strengths. Take care. Take great self care.

–Barbara J. Semple

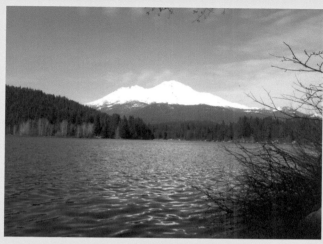

> *To see the greatness of a mountain, one must keep one's distance; to understand its form, one must move around it; to experience its moods, one must see it at sunrise and sunset, at noon and at midnight, in sun and in rain, in snow and in storm, in summer and in winter and in all the other seasons. He [or she] who can see the mountain like this comes near to the life of the mountain, a life that is as intense and varied as that of a human being.*

— **Lama Govinda**, *The Way of the White Clouds*

Introduction

Instant Healing—Accessing Creative Intelligence for Healing Body and Soul is meant to be highly experiential. When you feel ill or in need of uplifting, your emotions may play a role in your choices of support. Here you can choose a Quick Step emotionally by the healing names of each Quick Step. Feel your way along and have fun. Simply look at a picture and apply it to your body. *Healing Touch Quick Steps* may be easily integrated into your modern lifestyle. You are busy working, commuting, raising a family and life just fills up. The basic tension release routines called *Healing Touch Quick Steps*, many of them one quick step, are done by placing your hands on your own body at strategic, easy-to-reach "access zones."

You can do *Healing Touch Quick Steps* anywhere - in an elevator, in your car, at your desk. With just a little bit of time, 1 to 5 or even 10 minutes if you can, doing one *Healing Touch Quick Step* hand placement may help numerous body functions because you are tapping into your body's natural system of healing. The whole system benefits because everything is connected to everything else in your body-mind-spirit.

Having the healing power of Nature with a capital "N" at your fingertips is quite extraordinary. In fact, Nature is a visible, palpable expression of who we are when we get out of our heads and centered in our hearts of unity. Consider this. The word "natural" comes from the word Nature. The dictionary defines Nature as:

- The material world and its phenomena.
- The forces and processes that produce and control all the phenomena of the material world.
- The world of living things and the outdoors.
- A primitive state of existence untouched and uninfluenced by civilization or artificiality.

Well, you get the picture. Nature is huge, all encompassing, infinitely dynamic, and every one of us has access to the powers of Nature. This is important because you can influence your natural healing system harmoniously as well as harmfully. Stress is a destructive influence to your well being. For example, scientists have found that a person's high stress job permanently rewires your brain and literally impedes your ability to make decisions and have a sense of self. Losing your sense of self. Wow!

The body and our environment are explicitly related and both have renewable and sustainable resources available for wholeness. Nature IS wholeness. At least 25,000 plus years ago, our human ancestors believed in living life in accordance with Nature. The rhythms and movements of the Sun, Moon, equinoxes, four seasons, four elements, days, hours and nights intimately affected them.

Untold numbers of pieces of archeological evidence in the form of pottery, statues, cave paintings and rock carvings have been found all over the world, where humans homesteaded as well as from their patterns of traveling for the best grazing and other clues to their daily human activities. Our human ancestors considered the life giving cycles of Nature sacred.

People have been touching points on the body for the purpose of enhancing well being for a very long time. With an emphasis of putting yourself in accord with Nature, here are some examples of actual evidence our ancestors helped themselves with healing touch as far back as 25,000 BCE.

> " *Nature is the one place where miracles not only happen, but happen all the time.*"
>
> **–Thomas Wolfe**

> *...our ancestors have taught us that we are all related, that there is a great web of interconnectedness throughout the cosmos. Likewise, in quantum physics the concept of non-locality shows that an event happening to one part of a system can instantly affect another, seemingly unconnected part. Though separated by great distances, quantum systems 'act like an intimately connected whole, regardless of whether their parts are far removed from each other.*
>
> **–Nan Moss and David Corbin,** *Weather Shamanism*

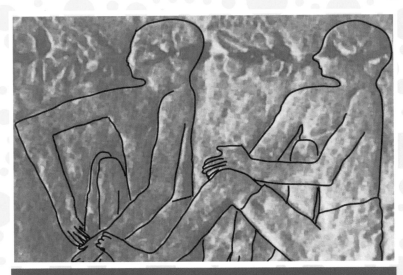

Drawing of Ancient Egyptian scene appears from a tomb wall from the Sixth Dynasty (2345-2181 BCE).

One example is a carving on a tombstone from the Tang Dynasty based on an early written text called the Nei Ching in the time of the Yellow Emperor (2697-2596 BCE) that depicts an inner landscape of the human body and speaks to touching specific points on the body as medicine relative to this inner landscape.

Above is an Ancient Egyptian medicine scene from a tomb wall from the Sixth Dynasty (2345-2181 BCE) showing a person and his friend giving themselves self-help by placing one hand on the inside of a knee and another hand on the outside top of the other foot.

I first found a picture of this in the book *Ancient Egyptian Medicine* by John F. Dunn, in which he says: *"The phrase 'placing the hand' recurs so frequently in the medical papyri that it seems to be the hallmark of an ancient Egyptian doctor, as does the carrying of a stethoscope today."*

The words on the tomb wall depicted in this drawing of "self-help" say: *"Make these give strength;" "Done to be praised by you, sovereign."* And, *"Do not cause pain to these."*

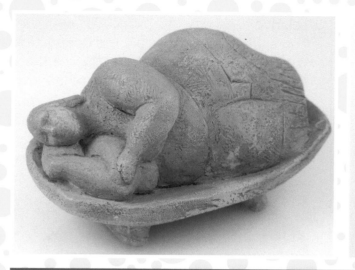 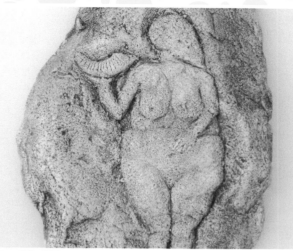

(Left) Reclining Goddess from Malta, 3,000 BCE. (Right) Goddess of Laussel, circa 25,000 BCE. Photos: T. Semple.

Another example specifically of therapeutic touch as healing wisdom applied by our ancestors is one of many small clay statues found in a cave on the island of Malta near Sicily dating back to 3,000 BCE showing a woman lying on her right side with one hand on the back of her head and the other on her elbow in a sleeping pose that Tibetans have used to induce dreaming.

One of the most remarkable findings of a human being aligning her body with Nature is a carving at the entrance to a cave in Laussel, France of a woman with one hand on her abdomen, while holding an animal horn with 13 notches etched into it in her other hand, explaining her body's relationship to the 13 moons of an annual lunar cycle, the natural world. This carving is dated back to about 25,000 BCE!

New Science

Called "the new science" by some, this frontier science, including key members of the Institute of Noetic Sciences, is bridging science and spirituality. Expanding research on the existence of a Unified Field of Consciousness and suggesting living the Field with intention, including the power of prayer, and more is shedding unique light on possibilities for healing. A recurring theme of this discipline is that Consciousness affects you and you affect "It." The "new science" experts for example, are finding that Earth's energies directly affect our cell membranes, and that in addition to being influenced by normal rhythms of light and darkness, we are even more affected by electromagnetic waves (EMFs) of energies and geo (earth) magnetic vibrations. Humans do better overall energetically when Earth's magnetic movements are calm, and, Earth is not always calm.

Did you know that in any given moment somewhere around the globe some 400 lightning storms are erupting giving off electricity that vibrates in the space between the earth and its ionosphere? That doesn't sound very calm. There are solar winds and flares, even though NASA (www. science.nasa.gov, April 1, 2009) says we are currently in quite possibly the deepest calm the sun has experienced in 100 years and they are not quite sure what it all means. The solar winds are so calm that it is making it more difficult for space debris to naturally clear away. That's just one small piece of a very complex bombardment of frequencies with which humans come in contact moment by moment.

This is important because the new scientific data is one of the most outstanding reasons, in my view, for being in a personal relationship (through energy healing self-help, for example) with Source energy every time you think of it. Source is the One Constant in all of the universal, cosmic fluctuations and movements. James Oschmann, author of *Energy Medicine: The Scientific Basis (Churchill Livingstone, 2000)*, goes so far as to say that he believes that when we are in a relaxed or meditative state, the pulse of the earth takes over as our brain's 'pacemaker.'

These honorable "new science" specialists comprehend with reproducible results what mystics, saints, shamans, Hawaiian kahunas, spiritual teachers, poets, philosophers, writers, artists, and holy medicine women and men of many cultures have been saying for eons: "We are all interconnected in one web of life. What you do to one you do to all. To live in accordance with Nature is to know harmony."

There is an energy, a state of being beyond mind, beyond body, beyond soul, of "beginningless" beginnings from which all creation emerges and continues to be created moment by moment. This Source of Sources, "Big Picture" energy, the Silence, the Stillness, the One Constant of all things, is what you and I connect with when we apply *Healing Touch Quick Steps* self-help.

The Power of Nature in Healing Touch Quick Steps

In the early 1900's after healing himself of a terminal illness and then committing his life to figuring out just how he was able to heal himself, a Japanese man named Jiro Murai spent his time walking around Tokyo and all over Japan, visiting the homes of people who were ill, placing his hands on them, and watching them get well. A well-educated scientist and an avid student of life, Jiro Murai was known simply as "the Teacher."

From his 40 years of research including

> " Through our exquisitely woven sensory radar we are capable of far more nourishment and direction from the electromagnetic field than we now allow ourselves... use the light body [inner body] to navigate the electromagnetic waters which we call the universe. "

–Jose Arguelles,
The Mayan Factor

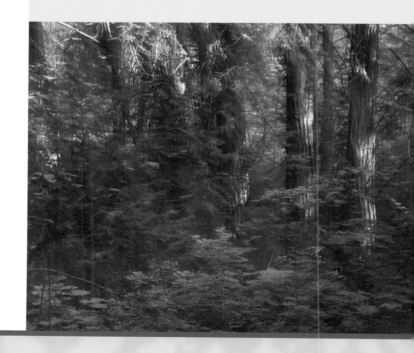

studying many of the world's sacred spiritual texts, Master Murai found common threads describing the relationships between Nature and healing the human body. Being a lover of knowledge and the intense scientist that he was, Master Murai was the kind of person who would fast for 2 or 3 weeks at a time and then eat nothing but rice to see how rice influenced or changed what he called the "natural conformation" of the body's energy systems. Then he'd fast for another two or three weeks and then eat nothing but fish to see how fish changed the body's natural conformation, and so on. Through his diligence, Master Murai refined and created the fundamental principles of what we know today as the physio-philosophy (Nature philosophy) he called *Jin Shin Jyutsu*.

Why this may matter to you, Reader, is because the *Healing Touch Quick Steps* you see in the book you now hold in your hands, are primarily based on the self-healing information of the art of *Jin Shin Jyutsu*® that Master Jiro Murai gave to Mary Burmeister as a gift to the Western world. A Japanese American woman, wife, mother, scientist, and pragmatic mystic in her own right, Mary Burmeister continued the research and teachings of Master Murai over the next 60 years. And now a number of her students are carrying on their own life research of this ancient art and the sharing of this extraordinary knowledge with the world.

Master Jiro Murai had the inspired foresight many, many moons ago to call this universal innate healing art *Jin Shin Jyutsu,* which he had "rediscovered" as having been in existence long before the time of Buddha and Moses. The words *Jin Shin Jyutsu* translate as "The Art of the Creator through Compassionate Man." I have further translated for myself the meaning of "Art of the Creator through Compassionate Man" as this: You and I can choose to compassionately tap into the force of Creative Intelligence that is the same within and around us, for our own wholeness.

What is Harmony?
I used to think harmony was two or more people singing together like the harmonizing music sung by the Everly Brothers, or a church choir.

Even if you are not sure what harmony is, you probably have a sense of what it is NOT. Feeling out of balance is the opposite of feeling harmonious. Truth is that in spite of all the disturbances occurring in and around you, harmony is occurring all over the place too! We exist in an ocean of harmony. Yes, "doo doo" happens, AND you have some control over invoking harmony.

Harmony of body and soul in any given moment may be different for each of us.

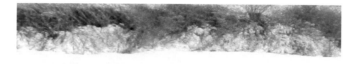

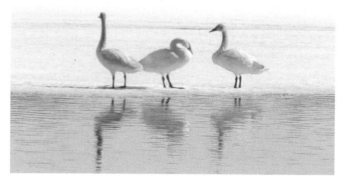

Harmony is that state of being in which you feel an effortless sense of ease, grace and joy. When you experience grace, you may notice your body-mind rhythms are in a comfortable alignment with Nature's rhythms. Nature is a most outstanding expression of Source (that Source "battery" that Mary Burmeister talks about) continuously animating and creating life. The energy healing self-help in this book brings you in synch with Nature's movements by connecting with Source "battery." When you live your life in accordance with Nature, life becomes more content. It doesn't mean "doo doo" will never happen. "Doo doo" still happens only now you handle it smoothly and gracefully.

Harmony is unique to you depending on where you are in your healing process. To you harmony may mean stress relieved, immune system boosted, muscles toned, elimination and digestion improved, circulation increased, or that often debilitating emotion called fear, disarmed. Harmony is also less specific. It can be simply a state of feeling your body and soul unconditionally loved in an uplifting natural flow.

So harmony is a multi-level experience that may be different for each of us. We are all created in the same Oneness, and how it "appears on the outside" is variable because of hereditary influences, environment, genetics, and any number of circumstances. It is what it is. You may not feel anything with *Healing Touch Quick Steps.* You may resonate better with another form of energy help like *Tai Chi* or *Qi Gong.* Your healing process and your destiny are yours alone. That's why I encourage you to always look for *your* harmony and balance. Compare yourself only to you. Be your own testimonial of health.

"May help harmonize"

The word "harmony" from the dictionary, means *agreement; accord; a consistent, orderly or pleasing arrangement of parts; congruity.* Since harmony can mean that numerous parts, relationships, and interactions are all getting along well together, then "harmonizing" is an activity or movement of energy that causes accordance or a pleasing arrangement of parts to exist.

You have billions of interactions and relationships taking place within your body as well as your outer world every second. On the "outer," relationships with family, friends, pets, environment where you live, as well as your thoughts, feelings and actions all need to comfortably "get along with one another" for you to experience a sense of balance or stability in any given moment. On the "inner," your body has 50 to a hundred trillion individual cells, thousands and thousands of special body tasks and unique organ function details that are all living in an interconnected "community" and basically relating pretty well together.

In this book you will find wording that says that a *Healing Touch Quick Step* "may help harmonize" a specific symptom or body message. "May help harmonize" means that the Quick Step is helping to bring that health concern into what is its natural, whole state of being for your body, mind and spirit, in any given moment - whatever that is for you. You know, there are people who might say a day without pain is harmony for them.

When a "body message" or symptom persists even after you've given yourself self-help and you've seen your practitioner and your medical professional, most surely the body is saying, *"I need more help than this."* Your mission is to keep your body's environment as healthy as possible. Accepting the healing remedies from wherever they can come, including Western medicine or emergency care are equally as valuable as your commitment to urging your body to come into wholeness.

Tortoise gets there less frazzled...

Vast numbers of individuals think they need to race or struggle to become successful, right? Would it be okay with you if you could achieve the same results or better effortlessly?

Healing Touch Quick Steps may help get you there. Consider living without being bound by stress. This is an important concept because it does not mean you will be free from difficulties and challenges or that nothing will ever go wrong. Things may still go wrong and now you handle it all in the moment like water sliding off a duck's back elegantly with the confidence that you always have powerful things you can do instantly, anywhere, anytime to cause a return to harmony.

In discussing the concept of a "pain body" Eckhart Tolle tells a story of two ducks fighting. In his book *A New Earth: Awakening Your Life's Purpose,* two ducks are fighting. After the short fight is over, the two ducks separate and float off in opposite directions. Each duck will flap its wings vigorously to release any excess energy and then float off as if nothing ever happened. Tolle goes on to say that if the duck had a human mind it would keep the fighting alive by thinking and story-telling.

Healing Touch Quick Steps are beneficial like water sliding off a duck's back because they help you stay connected to your inner body, instant healing, Higher Self. Some place beyond the mind, your body instantly shifts from the messages it is given. Giving yourself a *Healing Touch Quick Step* is giving your body a visceral message. Your fingertips set the healing

message in motion. You are not negating or pushing down an emotional feeling. You are being present as an observer from your wholeness level of awareness, while the emotional disturbance is occurring.

Like the duck that flapped its wings and went on its way as if nothing had happened, so may you move on your merry way as if nothing had happened as the emotional, physical, mental or whatever energy disturbance is complete. You have returned within yourself to what feels neutral. You might say that giving yourself *Healing Touch Quick Steps* is active "wing flapping!"

Challenges transformed
Think about your life challenges right now. Imagine now the power in your hands to affect your own healing. You are fully present in your life. You can problem solve really effortlessly. Time in your day suddenly expands. You have more time. You are more productive.

You are in a flow. Your zest for life is stronger. Opportunities start to open up for you. Your body starts working as a powerful teammate. People don't necessarily come to *Healing Touch Quick Steps* as a fountain of youth, and they are so surprised when they do look younger after a session or self-help routine. You may look younger, with more sparkle in your eyes and you are able to maintain higher energy levels because you are literally jumpstarting your healthy Infinite Life-Force unobstructed, forward motion flow. This is so important because the Cosmic Life Force that flows through you is much bigger and infinitely more powerful than any stress! All goodness is possible when you tap into your body's natural healing system.

"I am the Star. I am the Planet. I am the Cosmos."
- **Mary Burmeister**

What are Healing Touch Quick Steps?

Healing Touch Quick Steps are easy hand and finger placements for connecting to "access zones" along energy pathways that feed life force into every cell of your body. These access zones are Big Picture areas connecting with all layers of your being. The

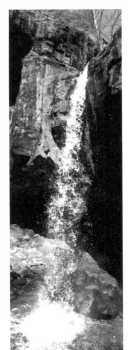

most important thing to remember about the places on your body where you apply *Healing Touch Quick Steps* is that these "access zones" are a direct line to your body's natural healing system.

Do you have problems sleeping at night? Your infinite life force energy naturally flows vertically down the front of your body and up the back of your body in One Big Circle of universal life force flow. This is important because if your busy *monkey mind*, to use a yoga term, is keeping you awake at night, doing a Quick Step may clear the mind by actively engaging your natural flow of life force down and out of your head, enabling the body to let go and rest. Down the front, up the back. That's the foundational movement of your Big Picture life force. There is more information about this foundational movement of creative energy in the *Top 10 Healing Touch Quick Steps DVD* in the *Healing Touch Quick Steps HOME GUIDE*. Visit http://www.healingtouchquicksteps.com/HTQS.html

Digesting and filtering more than food

Did you know that your body has to digest and process thoughts, feelings and frequencies? Gary De Rodriguez, Neuro Linguistic Psychology expert says that the human central nervous system with input from the five senses is *"bombarded by 2 billion chunks of data per second."* He says we normally filter about 7 to 9 pieces consciously and the rest drops down into the Subconscious Mind. The fact that our physical bodies come into contact with that much information every second is pretty incredible. All of the incoming data that goes through your system unnoticed by you and yet unconsciously influences you is another reason to have a daily energy self-help routine.

Have you ever felt like you just couldn't take in another thought, feeling or piece of data into your brain? High anxiety and brain stress really can overload your body's natural system of healing causing it to be unable to filter and digest one more piece. You unconsciously influence your life force flow everyday. Lifestyle habits, stress, food choices, emotions, the air you breathe, and any number of outside or hereditary circumstances can perturb your continuous flow and cause energy to become stuck. The flow can't go forward so it backs up like a clogged drainpipe. That's when pain and discomforts occur. The bad news is the disturbance may stay like this and even get worse if you ignore it. The good news is that

by knowing how, you may quickly move forward into harmony again.

Say you have chronic migraines. When one or more of your life force paths becomes blocked, the resulting stagnation can disrupt the local area and eventually disharmonize the complete path of energy flow. You know that feeling of something starting out small and pretty soon you are totally debilitated by the pain. Similar to the electrical circuit breaker system in your house, if one circuit or in the case of a migraine an access zone somewhere in the area of the head, shuts down because it is overloaded, you may jumpstart your natural healing flow to open up that blocked area. Doing *Healing Touch Quick Steps* 5 or 10 minutes a day may help you eliminate headaches, reduce the need for drugs, increase serotonin levels, and live a more balanced life.

More of the Science of Instant Healing (Worth reading, by the way)

You have the power to influence both your own harmony as well as your harm. From your thoughts, feelings, beliefs and actions your body responds. This is powerful knowledge.

You really are the creator of your life whether you know it or not. You probably already know some of the ways that you harmfully influence your health. You can easily begin to resolve these habits.

With *Healing Touch Quick Steps* energy healing self-help you actively choose to influence your health harmoniously. Intention has infinite organizing power. At every twist and turn in your life you have the ability to retrain your body-mind. You always get to choose - destruction (example, stress) or creation (example, energy self-help) of health.

Science also tells us each of our hundred trillion cells is a hologram (whole picture) of our wholeness. The American spiritual teacher, Gangaji says: *"There is no difference between inside and outside, between form and emptiness. To cling to either is to miss the whole."*

The cover of *Science News Magazine* dated September 13, 2008, shows a human energy body as a field of cells and the energetic environment outside of that human body is made up of exactly the same cells. The picture on the cover of *Science News* is showing just what Gangaji says! Science and spirituality seem to be in agreement.

The heart of the matter of active instant healing is this. The nano-second, or less than the "hundredth of a second" that you choose, intend, think about, or make clear your will and desire to experience healing, healing is initiated. This is important because visceral body chemistry has been triggered to create that which you desire. One hundredth of a second is fairly instant, wouldn't you say? Knowing how to access the "Source of All Sources" perfect health, instant healing opens the doors to limitless infinite prospects for good health. Plus, the body's natural system of healing is instant healing energy because you and Source are One.

Personal Body Talk
From an invisible, infinitely flowing state of perfect health, your body's natural system of healing draws support. Your conscious and subconscious mind may tell you otherwise. "If so, why am I still sick and miserable," you might ask?

How are you participating in the discomfort? Do you have an agreement with your body to get as much work done in a day and maybe take 5 minutes for yourself? Your life is so hectic with a full time job, commuting, picking up the children, walking the dog that your body needs to be self-reliant, you say? If you have read this far, you may be planning to make some changes in your well being. Among other things you do to affect greater ease in life, you could make a fresh commitment with your body that you will give it some energy healing self-help, for example.

Your body is more powerful than even the fanciest supercomputer. The body *does* communicate what is wrong and *does* advise when it is regenerating and healing, as well as when it really needs attention. Becoming adept at listening to your body's messages is another one of the side-benefits of a regular practice of *Healing Touch Quick Steps*.

Of course, tapping into the part of you that is perfect health isn't something you do once and you are finished. It's an ongoing thing. By addressing your wholeness matrix, calling on additional universal, life force flow to help release whatever physical, mental, emotional or spiritual stress has "clogged" a pathway, you may feel the stress melting away while some place beyond the mind your body instantly shifts from the messages it is given.

> *Any sensory input – whether you hear something, see something, smell something, taste something, or touch something – changes the body-mind's chemistry in less than a hundredth of a second. If we know that, then we can choose the appropriate input to influence the chemistry in a favorable way.*
>
> **–Deepak Chopra,** *M.D.*

> *It is a single cell's "awareness" of the environment, not its genes, that sets into motion the mechanism of life. Just like a single cell, the character of our lives is determined not by our genes but by our responses to the environmental signals that propel life.*
>
> **–Bruce H. Lipton**, *Ph.D. Cellular Biologist*

> *Consciousness is a substance outside the confines of our bodies – a highly ordered energy with the capacity to change physical matter. Directing thoughts at a target seemed capable of altering machines, cells, and indeed, entire multi-celled organisms like human beings. This mind-over-matter power even seemed to traverse space and time. The evidence suggests that human thoughts and intentions are an actual physical 'something'… Every thought we have is a tangible energy with the power to transform. A thought is not only a thing: a thought is a thing that influences other things.*
>
> **–Lynne McTaggart**
> *Author of* The Field

The Body Knows Before You Do

The body knows best, and does tell all. The easiest way to discover what is going on in your life and the world around you is to take a minute or two and tune in to your body. Drop your shoulders and exhale. Look at yourself with compassion. Tenderly listen. Are you holding your breath? When you scan your body do you notice any places on your body that hurt, itch, tingle, or feel numb? Is there redness or puffiness anywhere? Do you feel tired or drained of energy? Your body is always giving you messages about what it needs to be in balance again.

The body is so magnificently intelligent that it actually knows what's happening long before you are conscientious of any symptoms. I'll give you an example.

Some time ago I decided to have a calcium CT scan of my heart arteries. Heart "projects" and the harmful beliefs about them loomed in the background and I wanted to be proactive in knowing where I stand. I do feel every one of us has the ability to positively influence our health and well being even at a genetic level because Source, Unified Field of Consciousness, Oneness is not bound by space and time or stress or anything.

Anyway, so I'm in the room for the CT scan. The nurse technician takes my blood pressure and it was 151 over 88. Wow, my body was certainly giving me a vivid message! Usually my blood pressure runs on the low side, say 106 over 55 or something like that. Immediately the nurse says your blood pressure is definitely a risk factor. I say, *"Give me a minute."* She continues to talk about all of the other risk factors to look for, and I have immediately put my fingertips in my opposite armpits. I begin to exhale while I am having a silent conversation with my subconscious mind. I say, *"Dear Subconscious, It seems that we are feeling really afraid here. Remember, this is only a test. I chose to have this done to see where I stand. It's okay. We are safe. Please let's calm down. Thank you."*

This conversation with my subconscious mind while connecting to my body's natural system of healing by keeping my fingertips in my opposite armpits took about 30 seconds. I asked the nurse technician to please re-check my blood pressure. She did and it was down to 126 over 79.

By having the presence of mind and a strong desire to improve something I was pretty sure I could influence, I witnessed a fairly instant harmonious body-mind response. You can too. A daily routine of *Healing Touch Quick Steps* may do wonders for your whole being. The happier you feel when your body communicates good feedback, the better your relationship with your body.

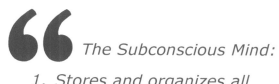

The Subconscious Mind:

1. *Stores and organizes all memories*
2. *Serves and follows instructions from the conscious mind*
3. *Uses and responds to symbols and metaphors*
4. *Takes everything said or heard literally*

What would you prefer to be thinking and feeling right now?

–Gary De Rodriguez
NLP Expert

Conscious "Languaging" is Good for Your Health

The names of each *Healing Touch Quick Step* in this book are healthy words you may immediately feel comfortable choosing as a connecting point for your instant healing. You may find yourself choosing a Quick Step based on the positive emotions you feel when you read the words. You are saying yes to your healing when you make a conscious choice of words or picture you choose for help. Yes, yes, yes!

It is literally much less stressful on your whole body-mind-spirit system when attention to your thoughts, words, and actions are non-violent, uplifting, and neutral. With all that your being has to coordinate on a normal day, when mental, emotional, spiritual and, or physical stress or illness are added, and Earth's geomagnetic energies are in flux too, the magnitude of your body's energy workload to stay in harmony is compounded.

Plus, the subconscious mind is a very precise "default" mechanism. Just do or feel or say something once and it is securely stored deep in the recesses of your subconscious and recalled forever again and again unless you change it. When you do your *Healing Touch Quick Steps* self-help regularly you may find yourself teaching your subconscious mind some new outcomes and responses to "remember" and replay again and again.

Author and cellular biologist Bruce H. Lipton suggests the cells in your body are constantly listening intently to what you think and feel. My sense is that speaking with "neutral" language is a good idea too, using words that do not have a "charge" so to speak. Choosing healthy words and imaginings in terms of self-help habits, instant or otherwise, may really amplify your healing. It's worth a try. The names of each *Healing Touch Quick Step* are healthy words and imaginings for body and soul.

"Unlabel" as Much as Possible

Labeling with words emphasizes a thing and attracts our attention to it. Consider, for example, scary medical disease "labels" such as cancer, HIV, and so on. How do these words influence a person's healing? Just hearing or saying these scary label words has the mind conjuring all kinds of pictures that may influence a nano-second response in the flow of infinite life force.

Your experiences at the sensory level that are *"unlabeled"* typically don't seem to intrude into your consciousness. This is really important information because when you can think about everything in life as simply energy that is stuck or flowing including any illness without labeling it, the hundred trillion cells of your body (and your subconscious mind) don't have to try to fit into the stressful picture, feeling and sound memory "file" carried forward from all of the people who ever came before you!

Avoid labeling or attaching to any serious illness name. Consider *"unlabeling"* and *"detaching"* from a diagnosis. You don't "have" a disease. You may say something like, "I am dealing with a health project," which is a neutral way of talking about a scary diagnosis. Or, "I am dealing with a lower back project" rather than saying "I have bulging discs in my lower back." Your language makes a huge difference in the success of your healing project. So, use neutral language as much as possible, "unlabel" and detach.

Return to neutral in your thoughts, words, and actions often.

> *Theoretically, if you were totally aligned with the cosmos, if you were in total harmony with its rhythms, and if you had zero stress, then there would be very little entropy in your body. Your body wouldn't age if you were totally synchronized with the cycles of the universe. If it did undergo entropy, it would be on the scale of the universe, which is cosmic cycles or eons of time.*

–Deepak Chopra, *M.D.*

> *We should treat the body as a faithful friend. If we spoil that friendship, we are in trouble.*

–Manly P. Hall

> *Labels lead to self-fulfilling prophesies.*

Marshall B. Rosenberg
Founder of The Center for Non-Violent Communication

1. Applying *Healing Touch Quick Steps* daily may motivate stresses to be released out of the mind-body system *before* they have a chance to settle in the tissue.

This is important because for your health you may want to harmonize a disturbance as quickly as possible, say, immediately after having had a surgical procedure, to bring healing energy to that area; or after any sort of injury, to bring an area back into its natural expression of wholeness, the natural state of your healthy tissue. What matters most about energy healing self-help is that you begin to use it. Look for your harmony. It's waiting to be noticed.

2. You get to participate in creating your own reality of health.

Traditional Chinese Medicine and the Five Element Theory address a "health-creating motion" for your infinite life force as well as a "health-destroying motion." Stress, genetics, environment, and your thoughts and feelings may cause harmful stagnation or blockages in your energy that are the destructive kind. This is important because by accessing "zones" on your body where tensions gather, you are actually choosing health-creating flow of energy *and* wholeness.

3. The more you pay attention to your body's needs and care, the more you may feel its divinity, its sacredness and wholeness.

By weaving your own path of self-knowledge while attending to your body's messages and symptoms in as little as 5 minutes anytime, anywhere with *Healing Touch Quick Steps*, you might come to know that perfect health is your true nature. If not, consider it research. Connecting with your true nature perfect health often, occupying your busy monkey mind with the application of *Healing Touch Quick Steps* self-help is a fun way to bring your outer world into alignment with your inner world (the perfect health, wholeness, instant healing world). That's worth a try.

Instant Healing – Accessing Creative Intelligence for Healing Body and Soul is all about *being* with your body's natural healing system rather than *doing* something difficult. The best thing about this book is the pictures. You don't have to figure anything out. When you are in deep need of healing, all you have to do is focus on your particular *"request"* for help because you are connecting to perfect health

Healing Touch Quick Steps

50

50 Ways To Love Your Self

Instant Healing IS:

1. A personal relationship between you and Source;
2. Your natural state of being in Oneness with Source, the Absolute, the One Constant;
3. A fabulous "seed thought" for your subconscious mind;
4. When you focus your attention on it, healing happens in a hundredth of a second;
5. Responding to life's "doo doo" gracefully like water sliding off a duck's back;
6. Saying "yes" to wholeness;
7. The more you love yourself, the more you care for yourself and the more Life seems to take care of you;
8. It's happening even when you're having a bad day;
9. Everyone is born with the same Infinite Truth, it's your choice to connect with IT;
10. Our ancestors have been connecting with IT for eons;
11. Infinitely loving, infinitely truthful possibilities for health and well being;
12. Ever-flowing, ever-expanding unified field of consciousness in which you participate whether you know it or not;
13. For some, IT feels like being held in the arms of a Cosmic Mother who says, *"You don't have to do or be anything to get my approval. You already have it. You are a precious part of Me. I love you."*

> *One part of coming back to herself [wholeness] is acceptance of her unique beauty... her soul shines through when she is being herself.*
>
> **Clarissa Pinkola-Estes, PhD**
> *Women Who Run With the Wolves*

Begin here – A through E Simple Tips

A. For fun, you may want to look at yourself in the mirror before you start your energy healing self-help. Then look at yourself again in the mirror after you complete all of the Quick Steps. See for yourself improvements and what harmony starts to look like for you.

B. Pick one Quick Step and kindly be with your body's natural system of healing for up to 5 minutes. There is nothing you need to do, really, except allow yourself to pay attention, listening with your fingertips in stillness without judgment. Remember tender compassion for yourself. You have in a hundredth of a second begun to relate to your body at a level of awareness that is deeper than thought or emotion.

C. If you are not sure how to simply "be" with your body's natural system of healing, you may occupy your mind by noticing where your fingers or hands are touching your body. Do nothing else. No need to dig into, manipulate or massage the areas where you place your hands and fingertips. Lovingly be.

D. Consider doing all of the hand placements for all of the pictures, one right after the other, for 5 seconds each for a quick **whole body tune-up**.

E. Look at your new harmony. Do you notice a healthier skin tone, reduced redness, sparkle in your eyes, less puffiness in your face, a sense of lightness in your step, less swelling in your joints or hands? This is your personal harmony. Very good! Very good! Yay! If at first you do not notice any changes, that's fine. No worries. The more you look for your harmony, the more it seems to appear.

> *Earth - In an endless cycle, the feminine as ancient and eternal as nature, constantly rebirths herself. Come, into the motion of the origin of all things. Come, be rocked and lulled by the Mother Deep. Remember to nourish her as she nourishes you.*

Field & Phillips
Wisdom of the Crone Cards

O - Complete Breath Hug

Fingers in opposite underarms

This is one of the best Quick Steps to do when you are feeling totally overwhelmed.

The Complete Breath Hug may help your circulation, the lymphatic system, breathing, any accumulations, and may help bring you to a place within yourself of total and complete - a very good place to be. This *Healing Touch Quick Step* may be very helpful for keeping the breasts and chest area clear of accumulations.

The Complete Breath Hug takes about 3½ minutes to do, depending on your own breath. **Cross** your arms in front of you and place your hands under your opposite arms. Your relaxed fingers will be in your armpits with your thumbs resting flatly on your chest.

Now gently **lower** your shoulders down away from your ear lobes, exhale and count 36 complete breaths, that is, one exhale and inhale, two exhale and inhale, and so on.

Focus on your exhales. Remember to **relax** your shoulders and arms as much as possible. **Breathe** comfortably through your nose and simply be present with your body's natural system of healing while you count your exhales.

The next time you are feeling overwhelmed, do **The Complete Breath Hug**.

When you feel nervous, or fatigued, or irritable, or you have a big test ahead of you, or you are going for a job interview, or you have to make an important decision, do **The Complete Breath Hug**.

While you are waiting in the car to pick up your child after school, do **The Complete Breath Hug.** When your child comes out, you are present, totally alert and there for your child.

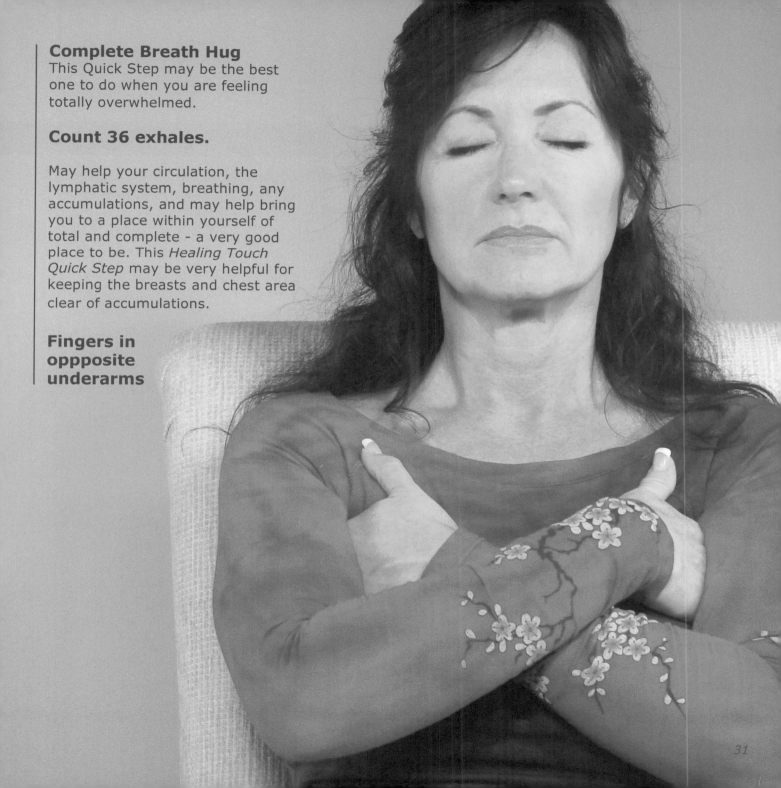

Complete Breath Hug

This Quick Step may be the best one to do when you are feeling totally overwhelmed.

Count 36 exhales.

May help your circulation, the lymphatic system, breathing, any accumulations, and may help bring you to a place within yourself of total and complete - a very good place to be. This *Healing Touch Quick Step* may be very helpful for keeping the breasts and chest area clear of accumulations.

Fingers in oppposite underarms

Maddie's story about The Complete Breath Hug

About thirteen years ago, I attended Japanese sumi-e brush painting classes with Master Hiroki Sakai in the San Francisco Bay Area. One day a fellow student, Maddie, an elderly woman in her late 60s with a number of health "projects," came to class and announced she was just diagnosed with breast cancer and would have a radical mastectomy.

I asked my Self in silence if there was anything I could offer to support her challenge. I remembered **The Complete Breath Hug** helped with any accumulations.

I asked Maddie if she would be interested in some gentle, easy self-care. She said yes. She had two weeks before going back to the doctor for the surgery. The doctor told her the tumor was about seven centimeters. During that two-week period she gave herself **The Complete Breath Hug** every time she thought of it—A LOT! She knew nothing about healing touch and had never practiced any such thing on herself. Weeks later Maddie returned to our class having had the surgery. She said that when she went back to the doctor for her pre-surgery visit, the doctor could barely find the tumor. It had shrunk to less than one centimeter!

Surprising isn't it, that something so simple as placing your fingers in your opposite armpits is really a major force of healing your body? Similar to the way regular exercise helps you over the long term by keeping you in shape, when you pick a few *Healing Touch Quick Steps* that you do everyday for the rest of your life, you stay in better "energy shape."

Then your body coming into harmony when you need it may be as simple as knowing what routine to do when.

Annie's story about The Complete Breath Hug

"The **Traveller's Aid Healing Touch Quick Steps** in your HOME GUIDE were extremely helpful to me on our recent trip. While on a tiny plane in Costa Rica shaken by the coming storm, I was not sure whether I would come out of this one alive.

While doing the **Breath Hug** I felt deeply in touch with unity consciousness. All the Quick Steps I did brought me into a deep calm state. It helped me to get tangibly in touch with this deeper dimension where everything is ok. It's even more powerful than meditation. Since then, I try to use the quick steps every day. The touching has a powerful and calming effect."

–Annie Reinhardt, *Business Consultant*

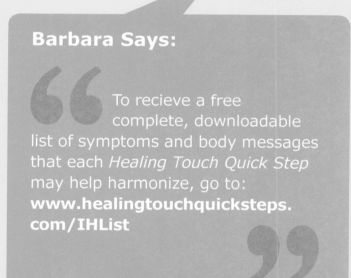

Barbara Says:

" To recieve a free complete, downloadable list of symptoms and body messages that each *Healing Touch Quick Step* may help harmonize, go to: **www.healingtouchquicksteps.com/IHList** "

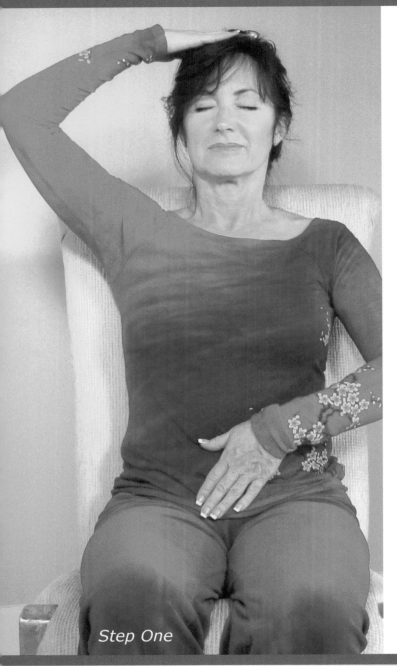

Step One

Step One
Top of head and tip of pubic bone.

Step Two
Left hand on pubic bone and right hand on coccyx (tailbone).

This Quick Step may be very good to do for any deep needs or critical care needs.

The Central Connection is a direct line with our Source of Life Force, from an ever-flowing heavenly fountain of Infinite Life Force; it addresses the energy flow down the front center of your body and up the back center of your body.

The Central Connection may help harmonize your endocrine system, is the foundation energy for all of the *Healing Touch Quick Step* energy pathways, and may help you recover your sense of self.

The Central Connection begins the forward motion that is the creation of health.

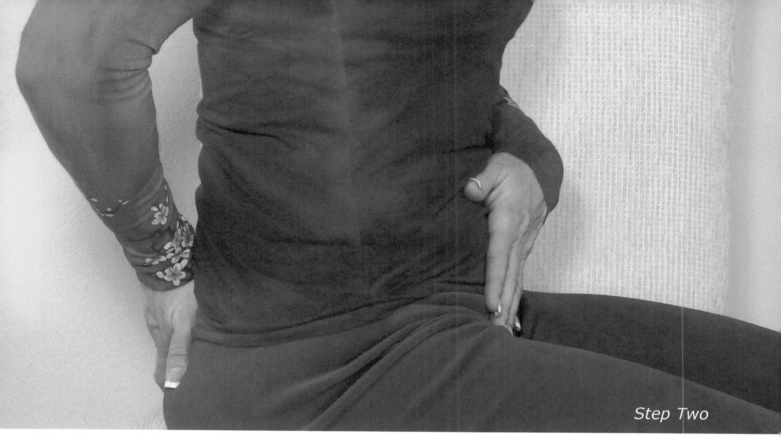

Step Two

The Central Connection can easily be done while lying down.

Step One:
Place your right hand gently on the top of your head while placing your left hand at the tip of your pubic bone.

Relax your arms, and hands and shoulders as much as possible and exhale.

Simply be with your body's natural system of healing for up to 5 minutes.

Step Two:
When you feel ready, **place** your right hand on your coccyx, or tailbone.

Your left hand is still on the tip of your pubic bone.

Relax your shoulders, your arms and hands and exhale, again simply be.

Give yourself another minute or two, up to 5 minutes, in this hand placement.

Back of hip and same side inside of knee

Higher Wisdom may very well help your exhale and your inhale at the same time.

The **Higher Wisdom** Quick Step may give your foundational energy a great boost. This *Healing Touch Quick Step* may also help you open to your inner guidance and can be very helpful for someone who is bored with life.

Place your left hand on the inside of your right knee.

Place your right hand on your right back side just below the waist.

So, you now have one hand on the inside of your knee and your other hand is on the same side of your back just below your waist.

Relax your shoulders, arms and hands and exhale.

Breathe comfortably and simply be present with your body's natural system of healing for up to 5 minutes.

If you have time, **switch your hand position** and take care of the other side of your body.

If it is easier to use the back of your hand on your right back side, that works too.

Again, relax and breathe comfortably for the same amount of time you spent holding the other side of the body position.

"Man contains within himself [herself] all that is needed for healing."

–Paracelsus (1493-1541)

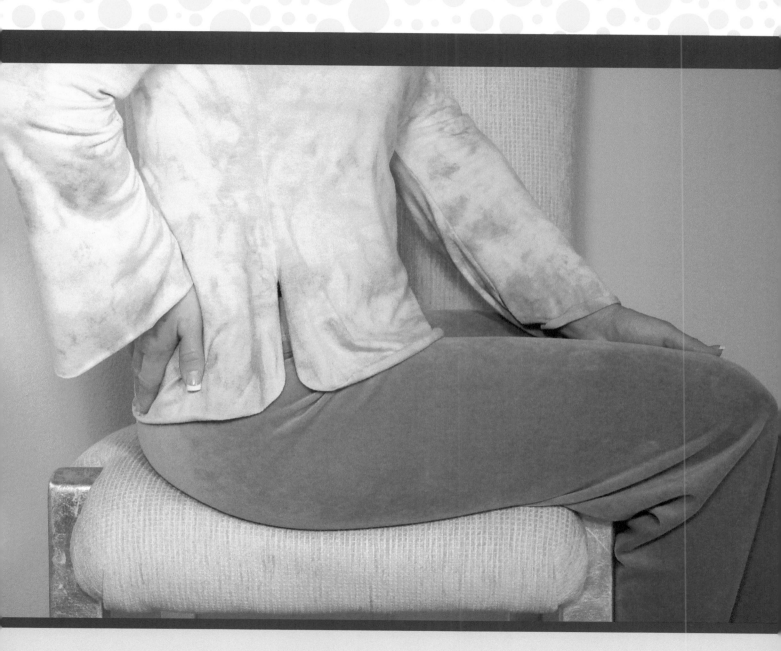

Holding inside of knees

The Great Movement may help get everything moving, energy, ideas, communication, any kind of energy that feels stuck.

Simply placing your hands on the inside of your knees is how you apply **The Great Movement** *Healing Touch Quick Step* self-care.

The Great Movement Quick Step may be helpful for leg circulation, and digestion, and for helping a person feel grounded on earth.

Place your palms on the inside of knees, either one hand on the same side inside of knee or you can cross your hands and place your hands on the opposite inside of knees, whichever is more comfortable to you.

Relax your shoulders, arms and hands and exhale.

Breathe comfortably and simply be with you body's natural system of healing for up to 5 minutes.

"The Great Fish Bone Movement"

One of my teachers tells a story about someone having a fish bone stuck in her throat at dinner. My teacher reached over and placed her hands on the inside of the choking woman's knees and the fish bone moved right up out of her throat.

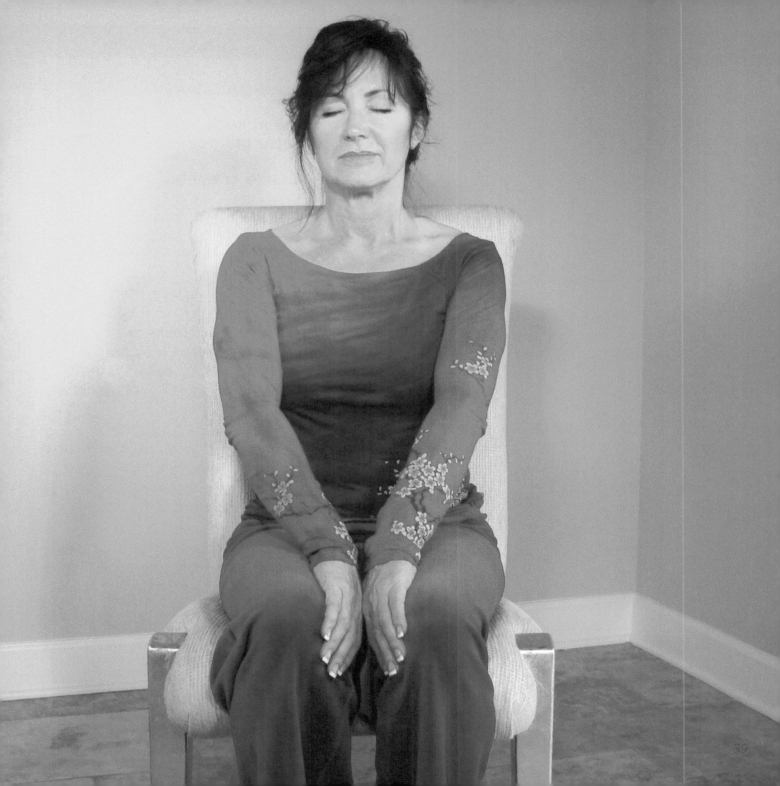

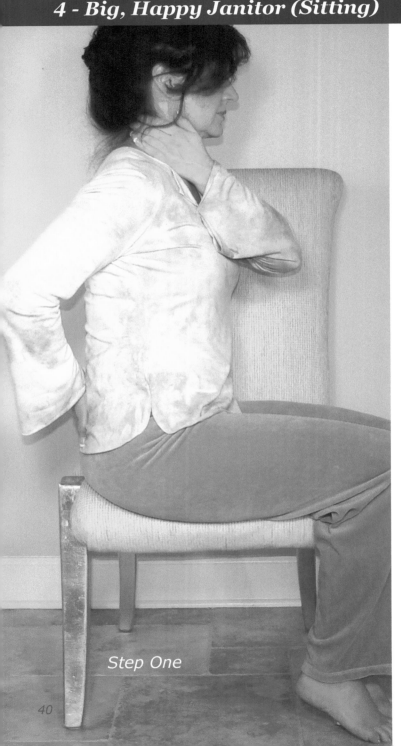

Step One

Side of neck and coccyx.

Then side of neck and back center of knee.

Then outside of ankle.

This one I do every day to both sides of my body. I feel it may be your very best "house cleaner."

If you take medicines, ever had numbing drugs from the dentist, or you need some help detoxifying any toxins or pollutants, the **Big Happy Janitor** may help release the residues from your body system. It may also help harmonize your urinary tract system.

The ultra quick way to apply **Big Happy Janitor** *Healing Touch Quick Step* is to simply hold the side of your neck and your coccyx or tailbone.

If you have the time, I encourage you to do the 3 part quick step, either sitting in a chair or while lying down.

Doing the longer version may give you even more help for a "deeper housecleaning."

Step One:
Place your left hand on the right side of your neck midway between the bottom of your ear lobe and your shoulder.

Place your right hand on the tip of your tailbone, also known as your coccyx.

Relax your shoulders, hands and fingers, and exhale.

Simply be with your body's natural healing system for up to 5 minutes.

Step Two:
Keep your hand on the side of your neck and **move** the hand that is on your tailbone or coccyx to the middle of the back of your knee.

Step Three:
Keeping your hand on the side of your neck, **move** your hand that was on the middle of the back of your knee to the outside of your ankle.

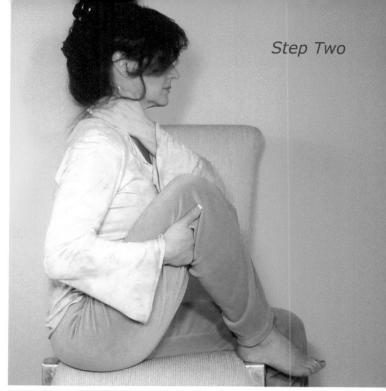

Step Two

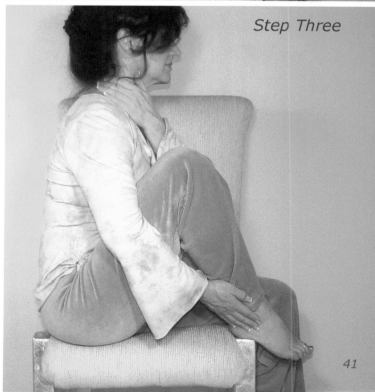

Step Three

41

4 - Big Happy Janitor (Lying Down)

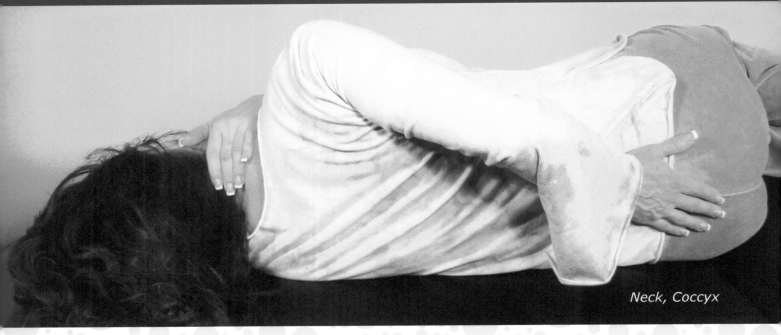

Neck, Coccyx

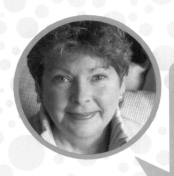

Barbara Says:

"This Quick Step may be very dynamic if you take Western medicines on a regular basis. **Lying on your side** while doing this 3-part Quick Step can be quite comfortable. I recommend lying down when you have the time to do so. It's one of my favorites."

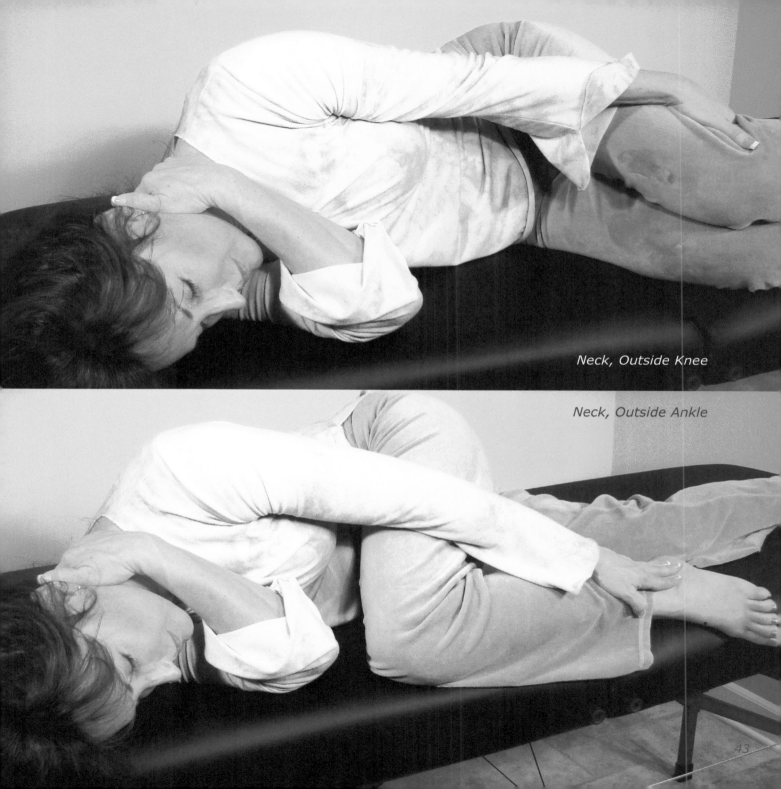

Neck, Outside Knee

Neck, Outside Ankle

43

5 - Gives You Wings

Holding upper arms

This *Healing Touch Quick Step* self-care called **Gives You Wings** may be wonderful for opening up the energy flow of your upper back.

You can't fly and soar with the eagles when your back is weighted down with all the things you put behind you, which can sometimes cause pain. When your spirit has been shot down and you feel constricted, you are closed in order to protect yourself.

Gives You Wings may help you open your wings, your shoulder blade area, so you may receive an infinite outpouring of abundant life power that lets your spirit soar.

To apply, cross your arms.

Place each hand on the opposite upper arm midway between your elbow bone and your shoulder bone with your thumbs on the inside of the arm and the rest of your fingers on the outside of your arm.

Relax your shoulders, arms and hands, and exhale.

Breathe comfortably and simply be with your body's natural system of healing for up to 5 minutes.

"Soaring like an eagle"

One winter's day I watched a bald eagle fly in front of us, flapping her wings as she flew upward until she reached a current in the radiance of the warm, sunlit sky. She floated effortlessly with her wings widespread without flapping once, for at least 5 minutes!

Soaring in circles, riding the wave of the air current without flapping her wings, I watched her simply "be" and I imagined her "being" in joy. The beautiful bald eagle disappeared from sight, still without flapping her wings once.

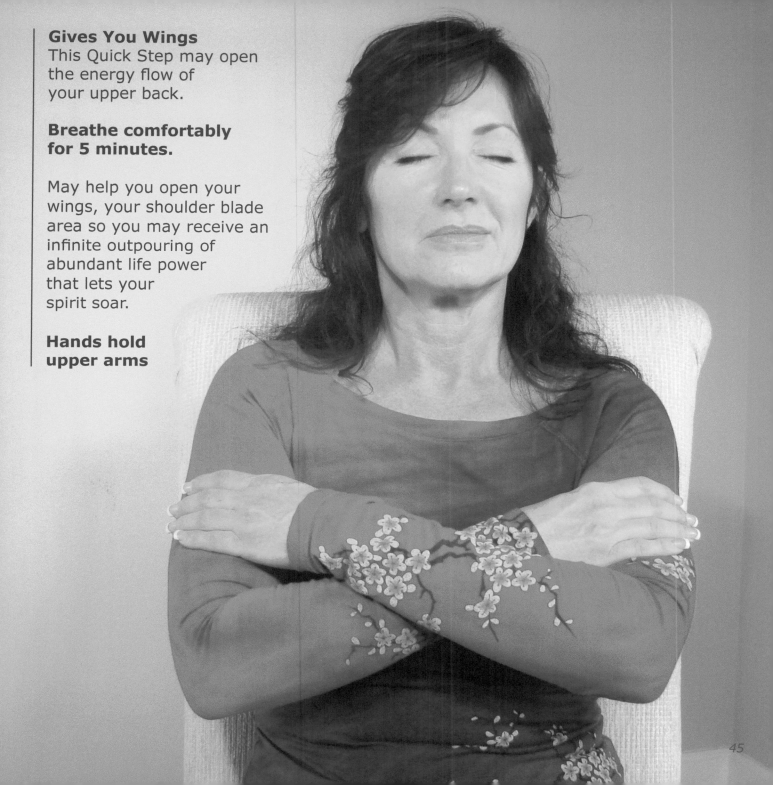

Gives You Wings
This Quick Step may open
the energy flow of
your upper back.

**Breathe comfortably
for 5 minutes.**

May help you open your
wings, your shoulder blade
area so you may receive an
infinite outpouring of
abundant life power
that lets your
spirit soar.

**Hands hold
upper arms**

45

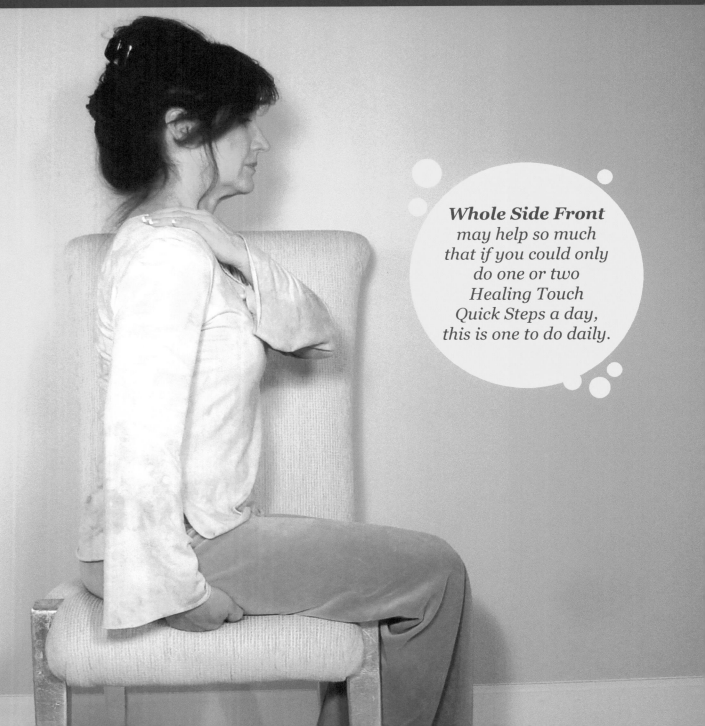

Whole Side Front
*may help so much
that if you could only
do one or two
Healing Touch
Quick Steps a day,
this is one to do daily.*

Shoulder and same side "sit" bone

Whole Side Front may help clear abdominal discomforts, and anything on the whole front side of the right or left side of your body, depending on which side you place your hands.

Drape your hand over the top of your shoulder, letting your hand lazily hang over the top of your shoulder.

Place your other hand on the same side of the body sit bone.

Your sit bone is located in the center at the place where the curve of your butt meets the straight of your leg.

Relax your shoulders, your hands and arms and exhale.

Breathe easily and simply be present with your body's natural system of healing for up to 5 minutes.

Then switch sides of the body and hold your other shoulder and same side sit bone for the same amount of time as you held the other side position. This *Healing Touch Quick Step* may be applied easily while watching television or even sitting as a passenger in a car.

Louis's story with Whole Side Front

A few years ago the heating and air conditioning guy, named Louis, came to check the air filters at my office.

He saw the massage table and charts on the wall, and asked about my work. Louis shared that his upper and lower back were really aching from working out too hard at the gym the night before.

I asked him if he wanted to know something simple he might do to ease his soreness. He said "Yes."

I suggested he place one hand on his shoulder and the other hand on the same side sit bone. And then, to be sure to do the other side shoulder and the same side sit bone. I showed him how to do the routine by applying it to myself.

Then I told him to follow up with doing both sides with the same side shoulder and groin area as well, for up to 5 minutes each step.

The whole process of showing him how to help himself took less than a minute.

As he was leaving he turned around and said, "I feel better and lighter already!"

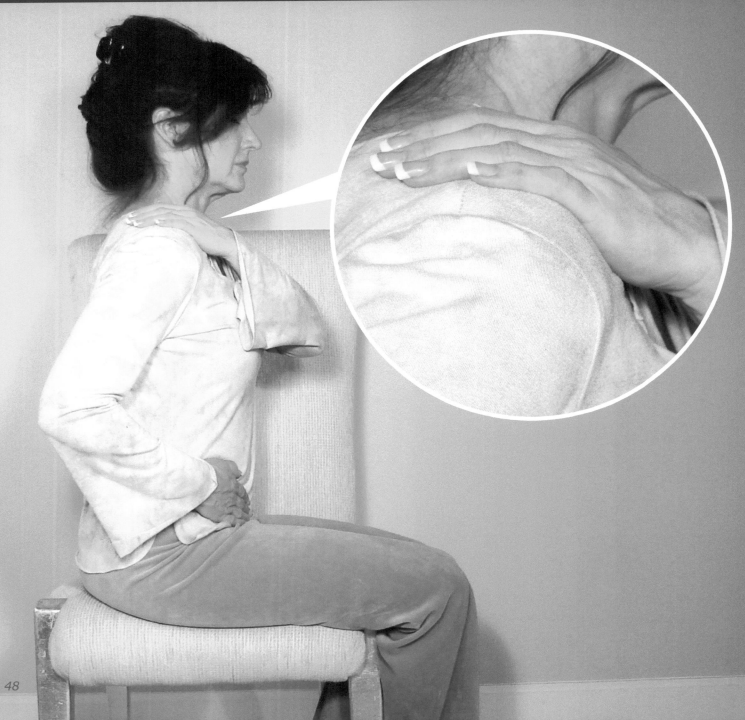

Shoulder and same side groin

Whole Side Back as the name suggests may help everything on the back of the same side where you place your hands.

Helping the energy ascend your back may help your breathing, as well as back discomforts.

Drape your right hand over the top of your shoulder, again letting your hand lazily hang, over the top of your shoulder, while relaxing your arm.

Place your other hand on the same side groin area. That's the place where your torso meets your leg. Specifically, if you have your hand on your shoulder, your other hand will be on the same side groin area.

Relax your shoulders, your hands and your arms and exhale.

Breathe easily and be with your body's natural systems of healing while holding these areas for up to 5 minutes.

Then switch sides of your body and hold the hand position on that side for an additional 5 minutes.

One hand will be on your shoulder and the other hand on the same side groin area.

If one side of the body is all you can do, that's fine. Doing both sides of the body is better.

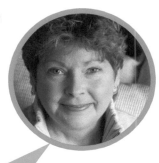

Barbara Says:

Doing **Whole Side Back** in partnership with Quick Step #6, **Whole Side Front**, is excellent for lower back discomforts. I've used this one many times.

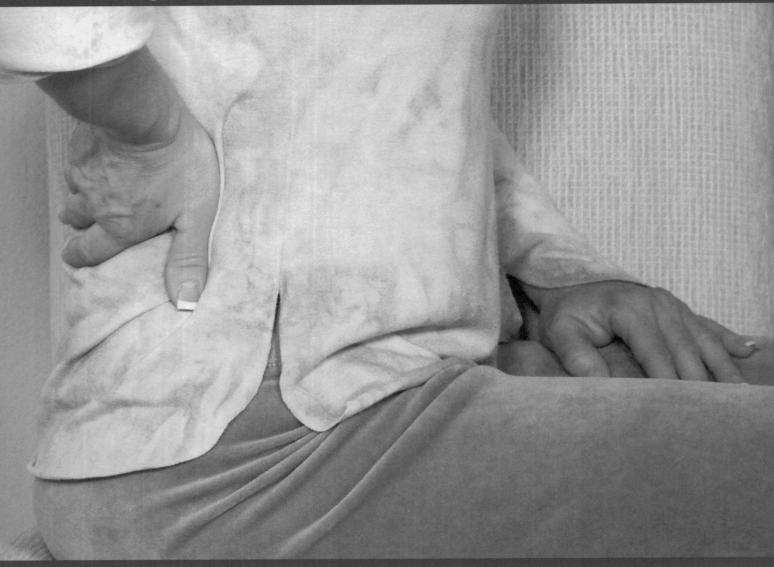

Back of ribcage and opposite thigh

Dancing Moderator and Emotional Balance may help with anything emotional. This *Healing Touch Quick Step* may be very helpful for elders, or anyone for that matter, helping them get in touch with their destiny.

Place one hand on your back side at the bottom of your ribcage.

Place your other hand on your opposite inner thigh midway between your knee and groin area.

Relax your shoulders, arms and hands, and exhale.

Breathe comfortably and simply be present with your body's natural system of healing for up to 5 minutes.

Then do the other side of your back bottom rib and your opposite upper thigh for another 5 minutes.

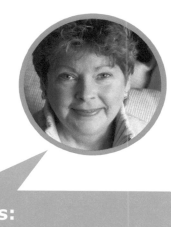

Barbara Says:

"You will find an entire audio CD devoted to **emotional balancing** in my deluxe HOME GUIDE.

Visit my website: **www.healingtouchquicksteps.com** for details."

Holding elbows at the bend

Completing and Beginning may help harmonize endings and beginnings and may help harmonize your personal power.

This *Healing Touch Quick Step* may also help sinuses, and breathing, as well as releasing the past without needing to know what every "past" is.

Cross your arms and place your fingertips in the bends of your opposite elbows.

Relax your shoulders, arms and hands, and exhale.

Be with your body's natural system of healing for up to 5 minutes or longer if you like. Every ending contains the seeds for a new beginning.

This one also works well with your arms resting on your desk at work.

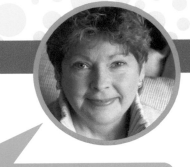

Barbara Says:

One reason **Completing and Beginning** and all of the *Healing Touch Quick Steps* self-care may help many different symptoms and body messages is because of the way your Infinite Life Force energy pathways naturally flow - intermingling, enveloping and supporting your various organs and all of their functions.

Your body is magnificently intelligent.

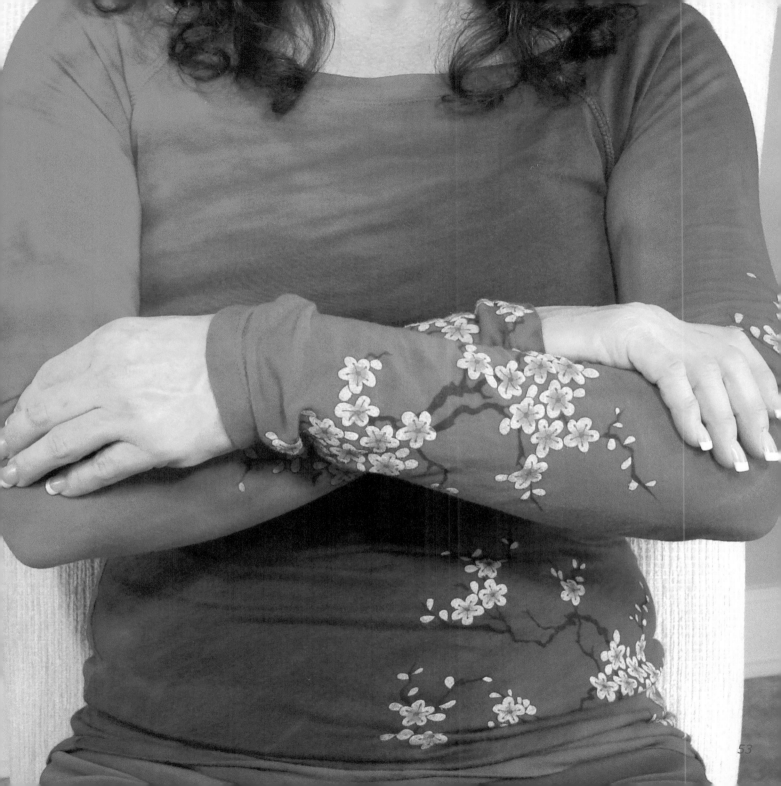

Groin area and same side inside arch of foot

Joy, Joy, Joy Quick Step may be helpful for relaxing the pelvic girdle, anything that has to do with your blood chemistry, and general support for the whole body. It may help the chest area as well as leg tensions.

Applying this Quick Step may work well for you while you are sitting down.

Place one hand gently, flatly, on your groin area where your leg meets your torso.

Place your other hand on the same leg at the inside arch of your foot.

Relax your shoulders, your hands and your arms and exhale.

Breathe comfortably while gently being with your body's natural system of healing at these areas for up to 5 minutes.

Then switch sides and do the other leg at groin area and inside arch of foot for another 5 minutes.

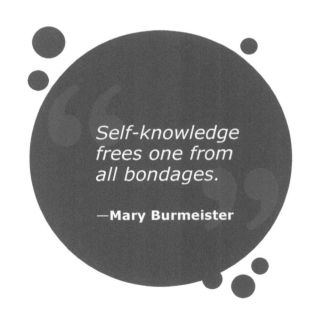

Self-knowledge frees one from all bondages.

—**Mary Burmeister**

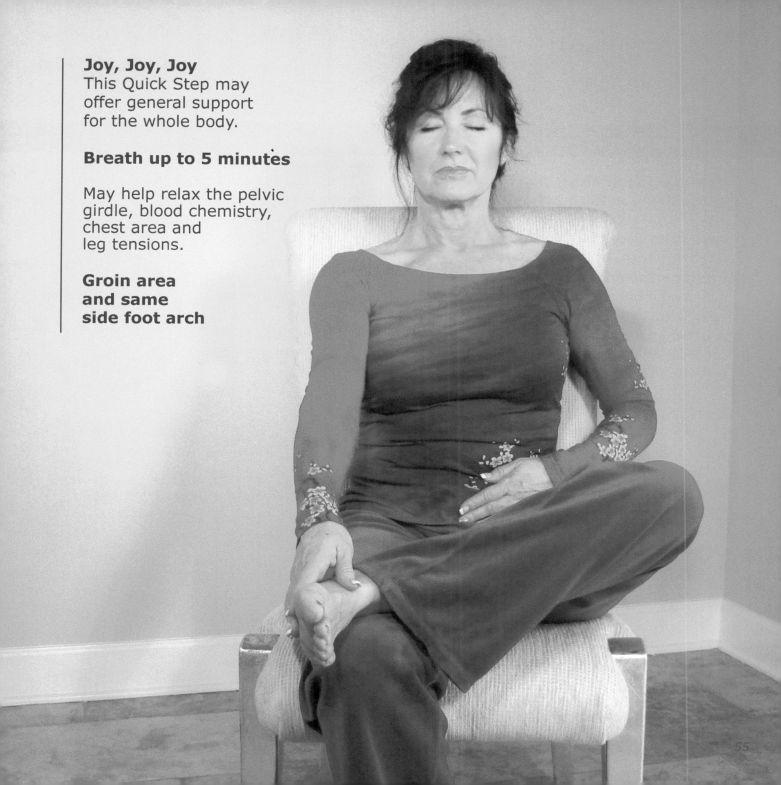

Joy, Joy, Joy
This Quick Step may
offer general support
for the whole body.

Breath up to 5 minutes

May help relax the pelvic
girdle, blood chemistry,
chest area and
leg tensions.

**Groin area
and same
side foot arch**

55

11 - Lighten Your Load

Holding side of neck/shoulder and make a ring with thumb and ring finger

Here is an excellent Quick Step for releasing tension and worldly weights from the shoulders. **Lighten Your Load** may help lighten your load of excess emotional or mental baggage or excess anything—too much information, too much television, too much socializing, and may be helpful for thyroid projects.

Gently drape one hand on your shoulder with your fingertips touching your back.

With your other hand, make a circle with your thumb and ring fingers.

Relax your shoulders, hands and fingers as much as you can, and exhale.

Breathe comfortably while holding these positions for up to 5 minutes if you can.

Then switch to the other side of your body holding side of neck and make a ring with thumb and ring finger.

Relax and breathe easily for an additional amount of time equal to the time you held for the other side.

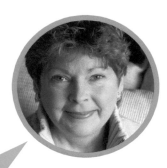

Barbara Says:

"**Lighten Your Load** may help harmonize all of the excess 'shoulds' of your life.

Isn't it interesting that the word "shoulders" contains the word 'should'?"

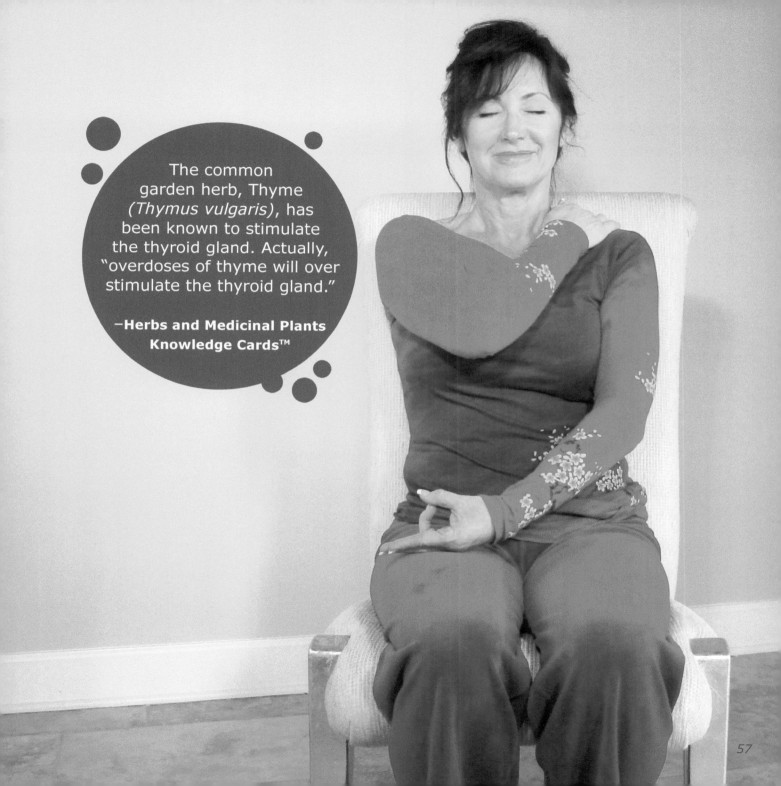

The common garden herb, Thyme *(Thymus vulgaris)*, has been known to stimulate the thyroid gland. Actually, "overdoses of thyme will over stimulate the thyroid gland."

—Herbs and Medicinal Plants Knowledge Cards™

57

Base of skull and opposite cheekbone

This *Healing Touch Quick Step* called **Eyes, Ears, and Balance** may help harmonize your eyes, your ears, and your balance, and it may also connect into the infinite life force pathways in the right amounts, according to your personal blueprint for existence.

Place your flat hand on the side of your neck with your palm resting on the side of your neck and your fingers touching the base of your skull.

Then place your other hand on your opposite cheekbone.

Relax your shoulders, your hands and your arms and exhale.

Simply be present with your body's natural system of healing for up to 5 minutes.

Then switch to the other side of your neck with fingers touching the base of your skull with your other hand on the opposite cheek bone for the same amount of time.

"The Weaving Princess"

Traditional Oriental Medicine speaks about a mythical *Weaving Princess*, who perfectly measures out the right amount of infinite life force to go to every part of the energy matrix that becomes you.

Changing your present does change your past.

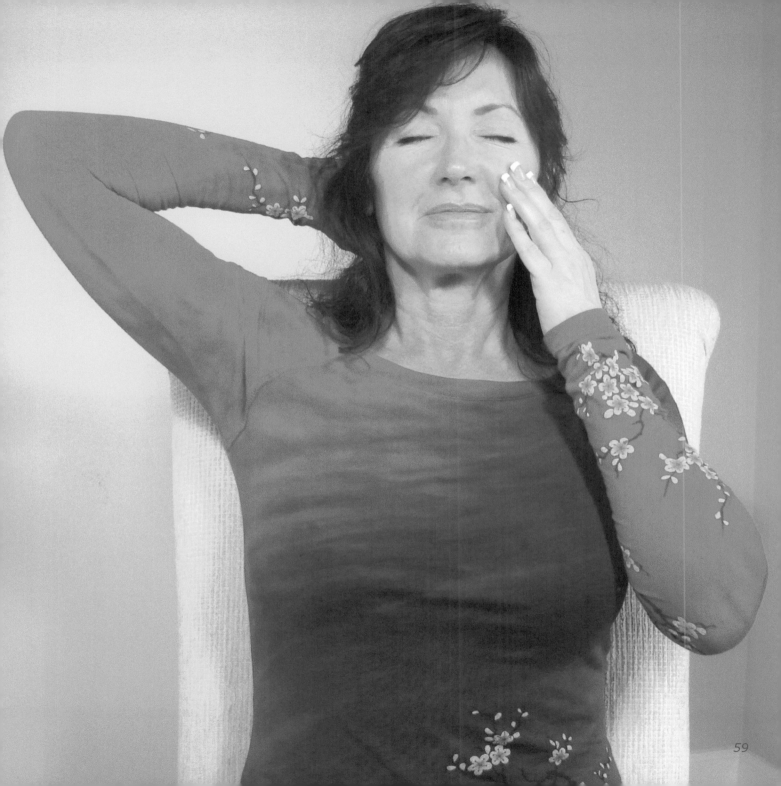

Holding upper arms, then hold each index finger and then each little finger

This one is wonderful if you use your arms and hands a lot. **Love Your Self** *Healing Touch Quick Step* may be very good for mothers- and fathers- to be, as well as inner children of any age.

Love Your Self may help you connect to your creative heart center, and universal mother energy.

Lying down or sitting up to do this Quick Step may feel very nice.

Step One:
Hold your upper arms. Cross your arms and hold your middle upper arms with your thumb on the inside of your arm and the rest of your fingers holding the outer part of the arm.

Relax your shoulders, your hands and your arms and exhale.

Breathe comfortably and simply be present with your body's natural system of healing for up to 5 minutes.

Step Two:
Gently hold each INDEX finger (one at a time) by "wrapping" your thumb and fingers around one of your index fingers and holding for a minute. Then wrap your thumb and fingers around your other index finger and hold for another minute.

Relax your shoulders, your hands and your arms and exhale.

Breathe comfortably and simply be present with your body's natural system of healing.

Step Three:
Gently hold each LITTLE finger for a minute each by "wrapping" your thumb and fingers around one of your little fingers and holding for a minute if you can.

Then switch hands and hold the other little finger for the same amount of time as you held your other little finger.

Remember to relax your shoulders, your hands and your arms and exhale. Continue breathing comfortably while holding each little finger.

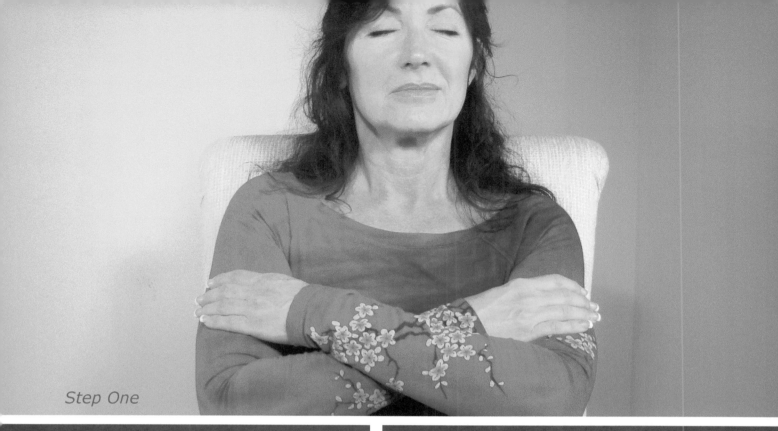

Step One

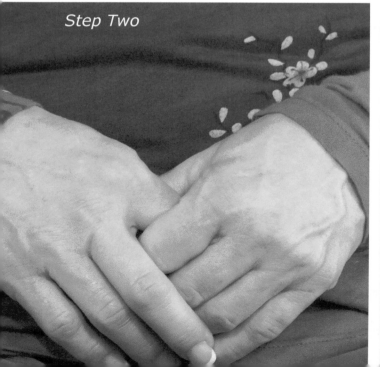

Step Two

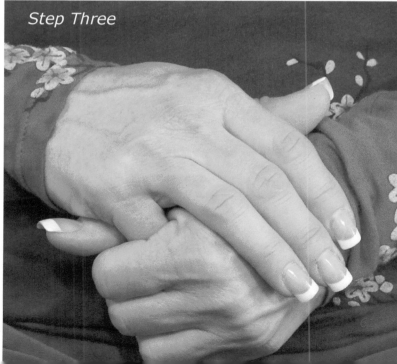

Step Three

Hairdresser's story about Love Your Self

Once I was part of a live panel discussion with a studio audience hosted by Vibrant Lives. While I was having my hair and make up done, the hairdresser was lamenting about constant pains in her arms when she raised them above her shoulders from the long hours she worked at this spa.

I asked her if she wanted to try some easy self-help. She said 'yes.' I showed her by doing *Love Your Self* on myself with her following my lead by holding her own upper arms and each finger.

Showing her how to do all 3 steps took about 2 minutes total. The hairdresser then raised her arms again. She said her arms felt lighter and some of the pain had gone.

...two minutes later, her arms felt lighter and her pain had eased.

Rosemary's story with *All Elements Come to Rest Here*

"I became very ill with painful osteoarthritis of my neck and an unrelated high fever. After two months I was mostly recovered but felt old and debilitated and had sharp shooting pains in my head and an aching neck.

"To my amazement, after only one session with Barbara the pains in my head disappeared. With subsequent sessions my vitality has been renewed and I am able to return to my previous activities.

"With **All Elements Come to Rest Here** *I have been able to relieve neck discomfort, stomach cramps, and the stresses of daily living. I will always be deeply grateful for healing touch self-help in my life."*

— **Rosemary Dyke**
Retired Registered Nurse

Oriental Medicine *Five Element Theory* explains the creative cycle behind all things human with the rhythms and movements of fire, earth, air, water, and the quintessence or key element.

These 5 elements have specific relationships with organ functions in your body. So *All Elements Come to Rest Here* may be helpful as an overall helper.

Paracelsus said that illness or discontent can only set into the body when two or more elements begin to work against each other. He knew that wars cause two or more elements to fight against one another, making a person's body vulnerable. Historically, it is after wars that epidemics have occurred.

Base of skull and opposite forehead

Then base of skull and opposite cheek,

Then opposite collarbone.

This *Healing Touch Quick Step* may help when you need a **whole being rest**.

All Elements Come to Rest Here may be very soothing, deeply supportive and restful, and may help anything in the head area, back of the head and upper chest area, as well as your ankles and feet area.

This routine works very well while lying down.

Step One:
Place one hand at the base of your skull.

Place your other hand fingertips on your opposite side forehead just above your eyebrow.

Relax your shoulders, arms and hands as much as possible. Hold this position for a minute or two, up to 5 minutes if you can.

Step Two:
Keeping your right hand at the base of your skull, **move your left hand** fingertips to your left cheekbone and hold here for another minute or two.

Step Three:
Finally, keeping your right hand at the base of your skull, **place your left hand** fingertips at your left side collarbone for another minute or two.

Relax your shoulders, your hands and your arms and exhale.

Breathe comfortably while holding each hand placement and simply be with your body's natural system of healing.

Switch hands and do the other side of your body when you have time. Doing both sides of the body may be very calming.

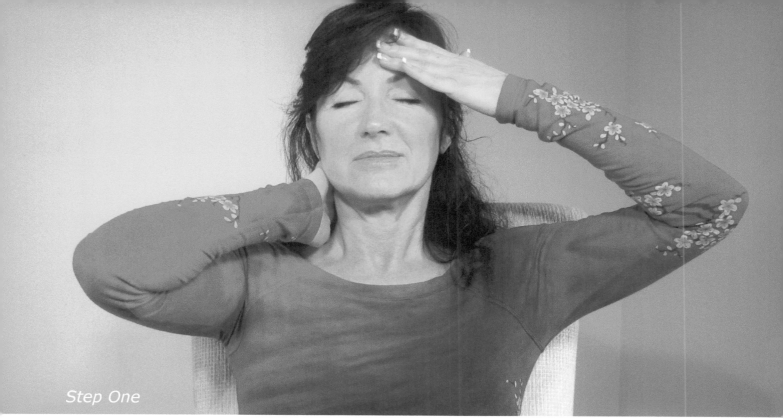
Step One

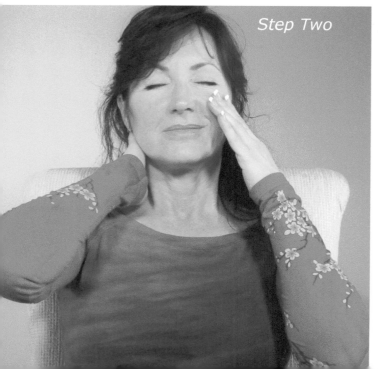
Step Two

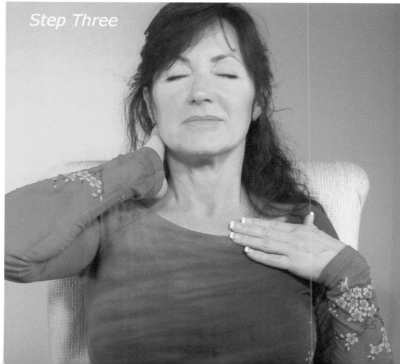
Step Three

Cheekbone and same side collarbone

Healthy Boundaries Quick Step may help a lot more than its name says. You can find a free, complete downloadable list of symptoms helped by each Quick Step, by going to: www.healingtouchquicksteps.com/IHList

Healthy Boundaries may help with all kinds of boundaries – emotional, mental, and physical - anything that has to do with your "personal container," which includes your skin surface containment.

Healthy Boundaries may be excellent for helping you get out of your head to relax and sleep, and may help with digestion.

Healthy Boundaries may be a natural facelift Quick Step.

Place your right hand fingertips on your right cheekbone while placing your left hand fingertips on your right side collarbone.

Relax your shoulders, your hands and your arms and exhale.

Breathe happily while holding cheekbone and same side collarbone for up to 5 minutes.

Then switch hands and do the other side of your face cheekbone and same side collarbone for another 5 minutes.

Remember, same side cheekbone and same side collarbone. Simply be with your body's natural system of healing.

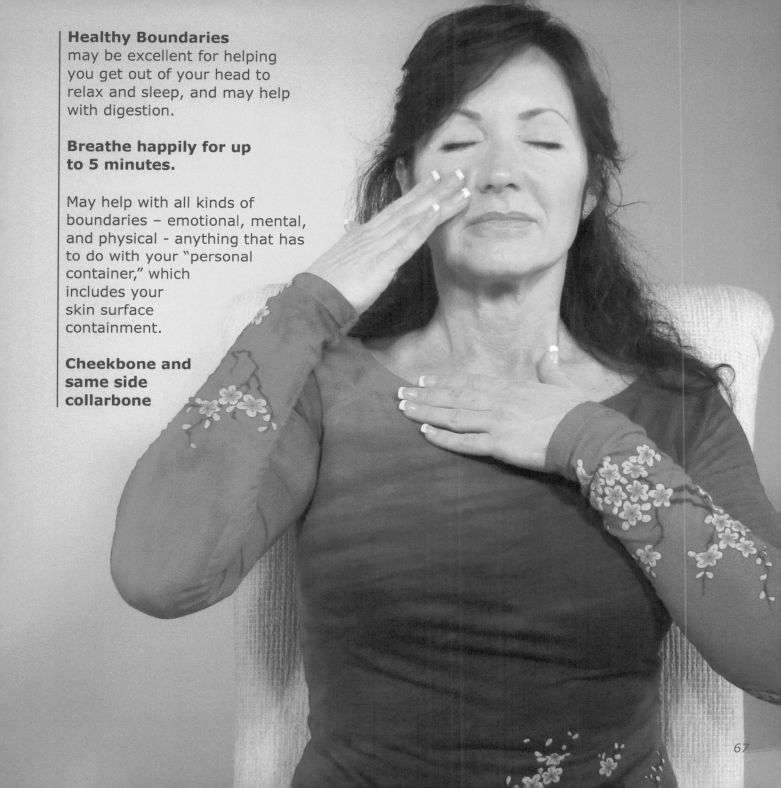

Healthy Boundaries
may be excellent for helping you get out of your head to relax and sleep, and may help with digestion.

Breathe happily for up to 5 minutes.

May help with all kinds of boundaries – emotional, mental, and physical - anything that has to do with your "personal container," which includes your skin surface containment.

Cheekbone and same side collarbone

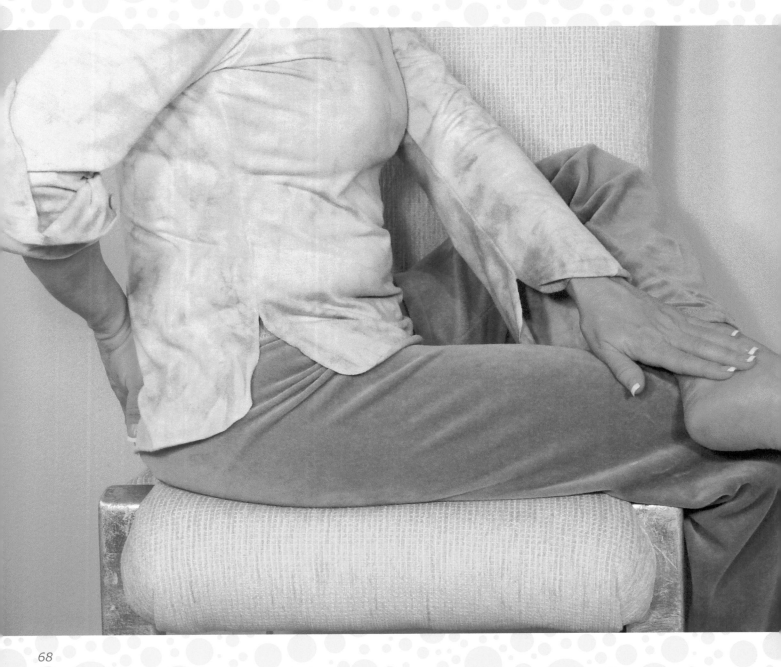

Inside of ankle and coccyx (tailbone)

This one is highly recommended when you are preparing for surgery or dealing with chemotherapy.

Nourish and Nurture *Healing Touch Quick Step* may help harmonize your immune system, white blood cells, and help your vitality and enthusiasm for life.

This *Healing Touch Quick Step* may help nourish and nurture your whole being, and may be wonderful for anyone about to have surgery or who is recovering from surgery.

Place one hand or fingertips on the inside of your ankle just below the anklebone and place your other hand on your coccyx, also known as your tailbone, or the base of your spine.

Relax your shoulders, hands and fingers, and exhale.

Simply be with your body's natural healing system for up to 5 minutes.

Remember, you can do the other side of your body for an additional 5 minutes.

Felicia's story about Nourish and Nurture

"I received Jin Shin Jyutsu sessions from Barbara every two weeks beginning with the second month and for the duration of my pregnancy, and did my self-help at home in between sessions.

After one session all of my fatigue was gone. I felt energized and elevated from that day on right up to my delivery."

–Felicia Z, *Mother of 2*

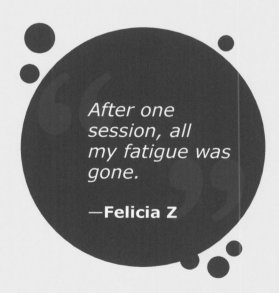

After one session, all my fatigue was gone.

—Felicia Z

69

Outside of knee and same side outside ankle

You can apply **Smooth Rhythm and Movement** while sitting upright in a chair with an ottoman to stretch out your leg. I like to do this one sitting on the bed with a pillow under my knee.

Doing this hand placement for 20 minutes on each side if you are feeling particularly achy or dealing with inflammation, pain or stagnation anywhere on the leg, may be very helpful.

Smooth Rhythm and Movement may be exquisite for overworked muscles, especially legs, knees and ankle areas, as well as helping to harmonize connective tissues, ligaments, and joints.

Now, with whichever hand is most comfortable for you, **begin by placing one hand** on the outside of your knee. Do this by gently holding onto the outside of the knee at that ligament there.

With your other hand, easily place your fingertips on the outside of that same side ankle.

Relax your shoulders, hands and fingers, and exhale.

Simply be with your body's natural healing system for a few minutes and up to 20 minutes if you have a serious ache.

Then switch to the other leg.

Applying **Smooth Rhythm and Movement** self-care to both legs may really help balance the whole body system. Remember to relax your shoulders, hands and fingers as much as you can, and exhale.

Barbara Says:

" Go ahead, prop up the pillows under your arms and legs for any of the *Healing Touch Quick Steps* hand placements. Make yourself comfortable and enjoy. "

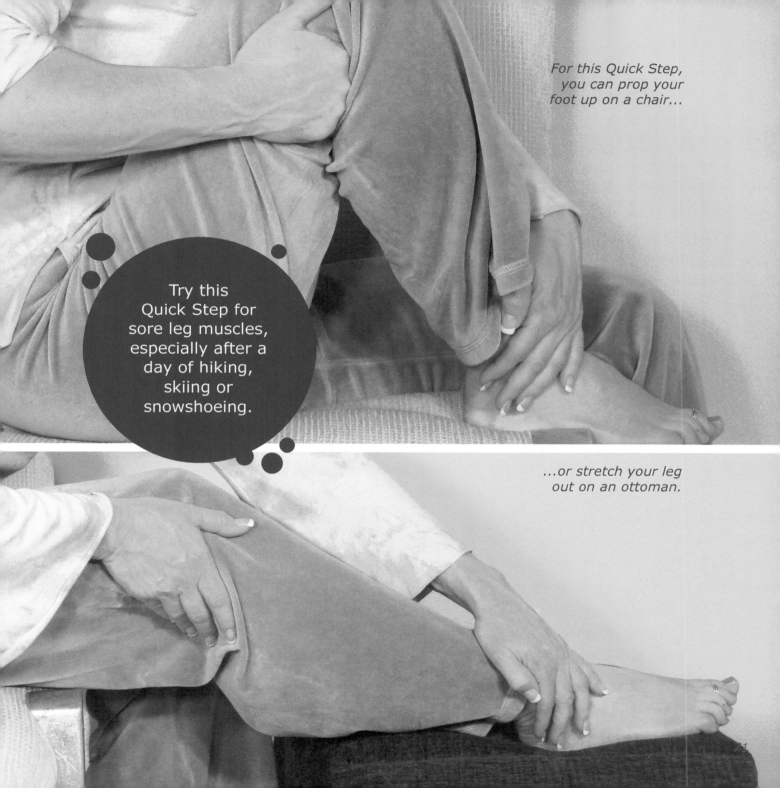

For this Quick Step, you can prop your foot up on a chair...

Try this Quick Step for sore leg muscles, especially after a day of hiking, skiing or snowshoeing.

...or stretch your leg out on an ottoman.

Holding upper arm and opposite thigh

Helps Everything *Healing Touch Quick Step* may help harmonize just about any need because it connects with all the layers of your being – blood, bones, skin, muscles, breathing, everything.

Helps Everything may also help balance the right and left sides of your body and the upper and lower parts of your body.

Place your left hand on the middle of your right upper arm with your thumb on the inside of the arm and the rest of your fingers resting on the outside of the middle of your upper arm.

Place your right hand on the inside of your left thigh midway between your groin and knee.

Relax your shoulders, hands and fingers as much as you can, and exhale.

Simply be with your body's natural healing system for up to 5 minutes.

So easy, isn't it?

Then switch your hand positions to hold your other arm and the opposite other mid thigh for the same amount of time.

Relax your shoulders, hands and fingers.

Pythagoras (580-500 BCE) taught that each person must attain integration of his or her soul for herself through a depth of commitment to and an insightful understanding of Divine principles which, he said, being scientific, are the same for everyone.

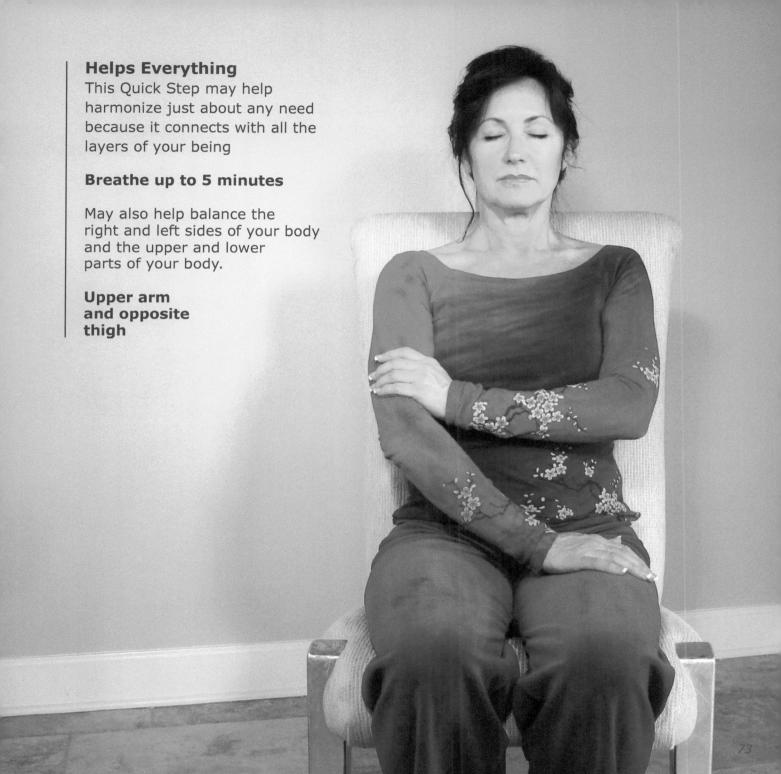

Helps Everything

This Quick Step may help harmonize just about any need because it connects with all the layers of your being

Breathe up to 5 minutes

May also help balance the right and left sides of your body and the upper and lower parts of your body.

**Upper arm
and opposite
thigh**

Sit on your hands. Really.

Muscle Tone and Weight Balance
may be really beneficial for anyone who is bedridden or spends a lot of time in a wheelchair, may help clear the back and help all of your body's ascending energy needs.

This is important because you are tapping into your body's natural system of healing with particular pathways that flow through these areas. The gluteus maximus muscles are the biggest muscles of the body. By helping your muscles you help your overall metabolism.

Simply sit on your hands.

The area you are addressing is sometimes called the sit bone and the gluteus maximus muscle is right there!

You can do one side at a time or both sides. This is good for helping your circulation when you've been riding in a car for a long period.

Please note: If you are helping someone who is bedridden, you can slide your flat palm under their body and then go to the other side of their body and do the same there.

Barbara Says:

" Weight balance is different than weight loss. Weight **balance** says you are at the weight that is natural for you at any moment. "

74

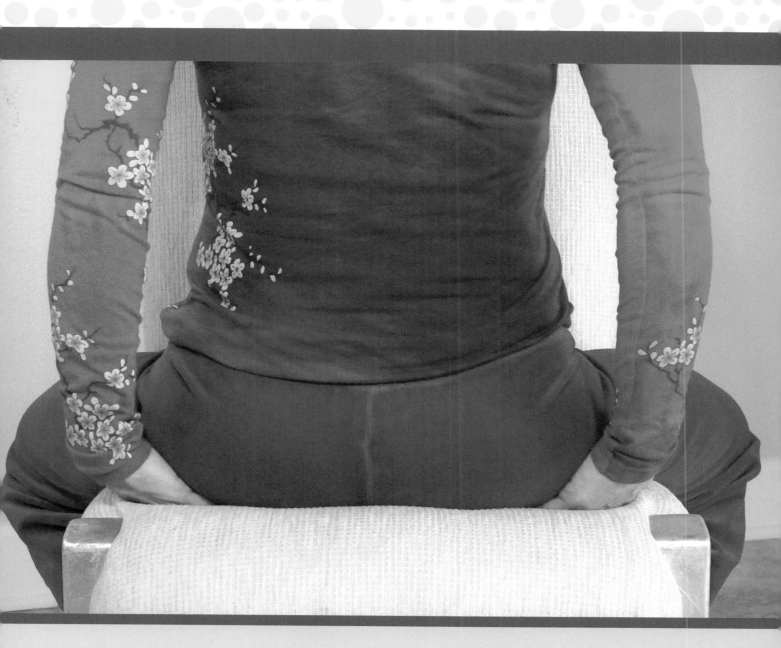

20 - Completely Receive

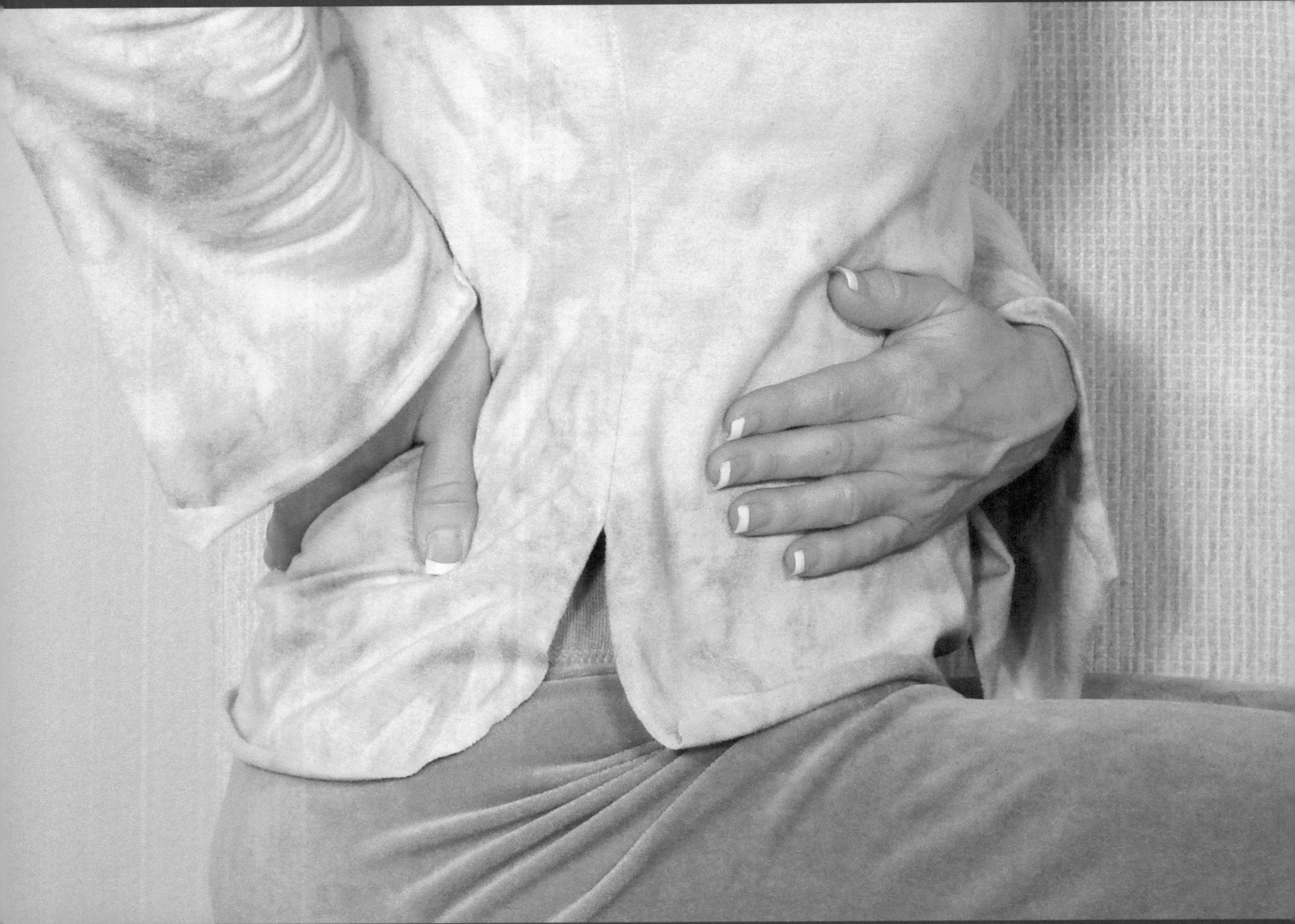

Palming back bottom rib and same side front bottom rib

Completely Receive may help the lungs, grief and sadness, and may help you completely receive the breath of life, the goodness, abundance and joy of life and love while harmonizing lung functions. Breath is important for the circulation of the whole body and may also help bring common sense to a situation.

Simply place your left hand at the bottom of your right front rib cage and **place your right hand** on your right backside at the bottom rib. So you are holding your bottom back rib and the same side front bottom rib areas. You may find it easier to place the back of your hand on your back bottom rib.

Remember to relax your shoulders, hands and fingers and exhale.
Simply be with your body's natural system of healing for up to 5 minutes.

Then switch sides to hold the other front and back bottom ribs as well.

Relax and breathe easily while holding front bottom rib and back same side bottom rib for another 5 minutes.

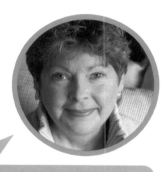

Are you dealing with a 'health problem' or 'health project'? A problem may be difficult and insurmountable. A project is a task, an undertaking that may be uplifting and seen to completion. Which sounds easier, problem or project?

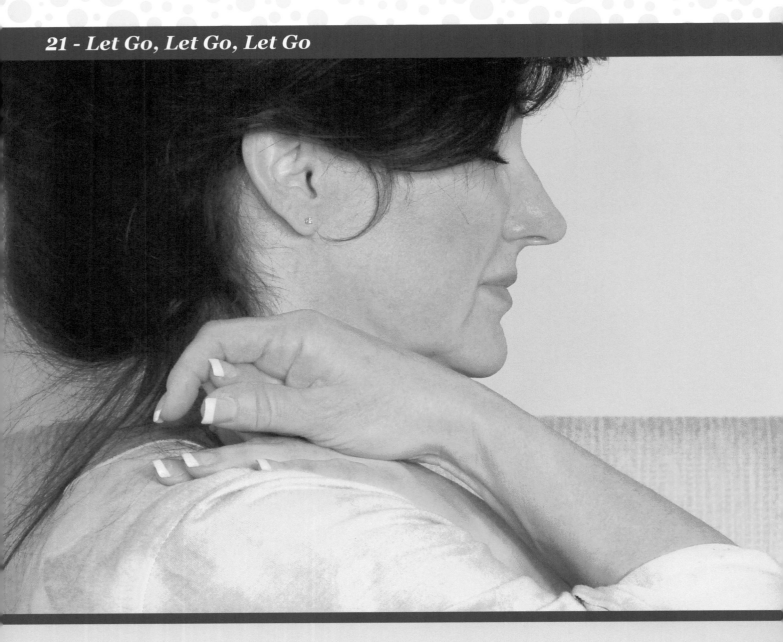

Holding shoulder and opposite index finger

Let Go, Let Go, Let Go may help your large intestine function, elimination projects, your ability to exhale and release deep hurts, as well as deep skin projects like burns, warts, or insect bites.

Place your left hand on your right shoulder.

With your free hand, hold the INDEX finger of your left hand, the hand that is on your right shoulder.

Relax your shoulders, hands and fingers and exhale.

Simply be with your body's natural healing system for up to 5 minutes.

Then switch your hand positions to apply to the other side of your body.

Jackie's story with Let Go, Let Go, Let Go

Jackie, a 60- year old woman had a fight with a friend she'd known for years. Out of the blue the friend became mean and judgmental of Jackie. Jackie's feelings were deeply hurt, she felt stunned, and she noticed that her side and middle abdomen had become painful.

During her healing session, Jackie realized that the feelings and physical pains were exactly how she used to feel when her alcoholic mother use to belittle and criticize her as a child, which caused her constipation and severe acne as a teenager.

As Jackie's energy harmonized, she was able to bless her friend and let go of this unfortunate life circumstance.

Holding at sides of collarbone

Comfortable Wherever You Are is a great name for describing how this one may help you.

There are two ways to do this one, whichever feels most "comfortable" for your hands.

Where you place your hands for this *Healing Touch Quick Step* is one of those major gathering places for tension on the body.

Besides helping you harmonize adapting to whatever situation in which you find yourself, **Comfortable Wherever You Are** may help you breathe easier, unload mental and emotional excesses - too many thoughts or overwhelming feelings, thyroid needs, and may clear the whole front chest area.

Place your fingertips on the right and left sides of your collarbone.

Use the center of your collarbone as the middle guide and then go to each side of that middle collarbone just below the actual bone.

Once you have your fingertips on your collarbone, **slide your fingertips down** off the collarbone to the soft spots just below the bone and rest your fingers or hands there.

Remember to relax your shoulders, hands and fingers as much as you can, and exhale.

Simply be present with your body's natural system of healing for up to 5 minutes.

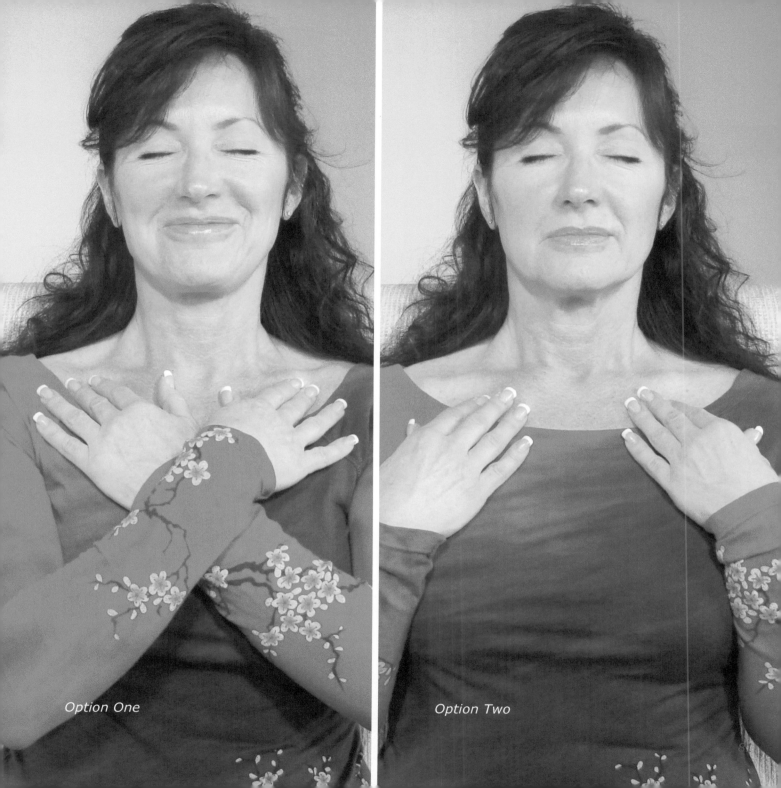

Option One

Option Two

Tip of pubic bone and little toe

Use Your Life Well may be excellent for kidney projects as well as all phases of a person's life, anyone in transition, babies, adolescents, elderly, and women and men in midlife.

Because of the energy pathways addressed here, this Quick Step may help boost the immune system and help someone with a critical need for healing energy.

First, cross your left foot on to your right knee.

Now place your right hand on your left little toe and place your other hand (left hand) flatly on the center tip of your pubic bone.

Relax your shoulders, hands and fingers, and exhale.

Simply be with your body's natural healing system for up to 5 minutes.

Then switch hands, holding the other little toe and the center tip of your pubic bone to help the other side of your body.

Relax and breathe comfortably for another 5 minutes.

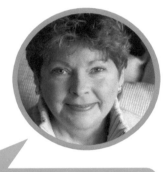

> *Filling up your energy reserves will give your body energy to correct itself.*

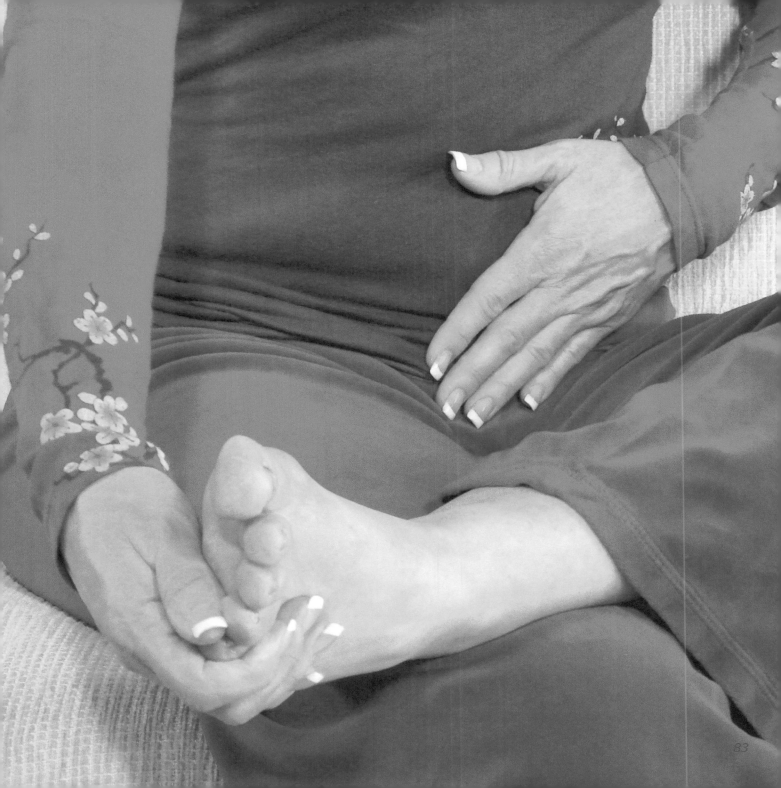

Holding elbow and opposite thigh

Have you ever seen someone who was barrel-chested and everything below the waist was super thin?

Or do you know someone who carries a lot of extra weight below the waist like being pregnant but they are not pregnant, and everything above the waist was really flat and thin?

Both of these people could use some help balancing their upper and lower half body energies.

Waist Up-Waist Down Harmony may help what needs to go down, go down, and what needs to go up, go up. That means this *Healing Touch Quick Step* may help harmonize digestion as well as inhaling as well as vitality and circulation.

Place right hand or fingertips on your left elbow crease at the bend of your elbow.

Place your left hand on your opposite (right) mid thigh.

That's elbow at the bend and opposite mid thigh.

Relax your shoulders, hands and fingers as much as you can, and exhale.

Simply be with your body's natural system of healing for up to 5 minutes.

Then switch your hands and do the other elbow and opposite mid thigh for another 5 minutes.

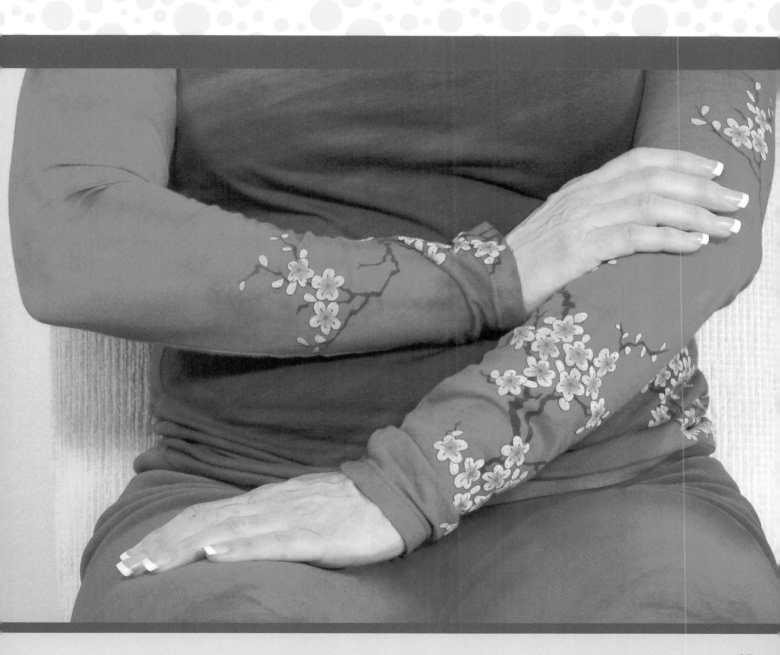

Holding big toes

For someone in the hospital or sick in bed, this Quick Step may be deeply comforting by helping the whole body breathe.

Breathe from Toes to Head may very well help your whole body breathe.

Simply hold your big toes.

Remember to relax your shoulders, hands and fingers as much as you can, and exhale.

Simply be with your body's natural system of healing for up to 5 minutes.

You can also see here how to help someone else (*picture two*). The same guidance applies when placing your hands on another person.

Remember to relax YOUR shoulders, hands and fingers as much as you can, and exhale.

Simply be with THEIR body's natural system of healing for up to 5 minutes.

Mother's story about *Breathe from Toes to Head*

Some years ago my mother was in intensive care. When I arrived at her hospital room she was unconscious with breathing tube for oxygen.

Scanning the situation I noticed that my mom's chest was not expanding with her breathing but her lower abdomen was filling up like a huge basketball.

I went to the foot of her bed and gently held her big toes. After about a minute of my gently holding her toes, she let out a big exhale.

I and everyone else in the room watched the big "basketball" in her lower abdomen deflate and her breathing came into balance.

Her chest and the upper and lower halves of her body seemed to be breathing normally from that point on.

I am always in awe of how simple and profound these Healing Touch Quick Steps are.

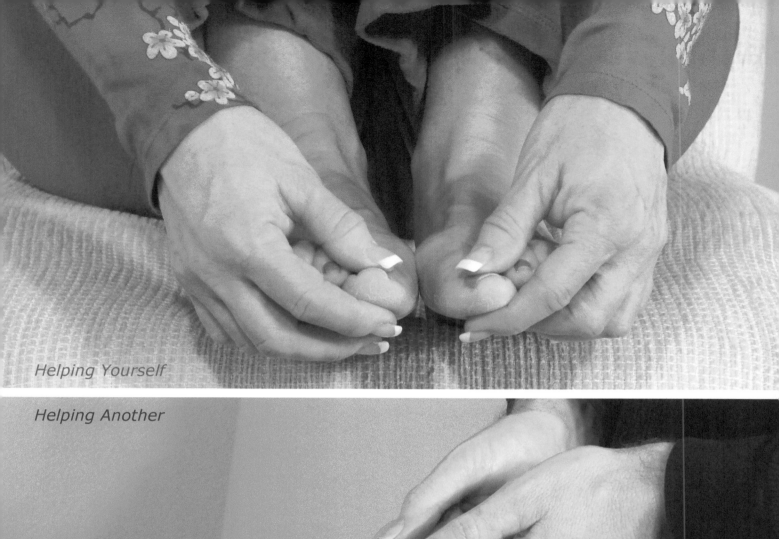

Helping Yourself

Helping Another

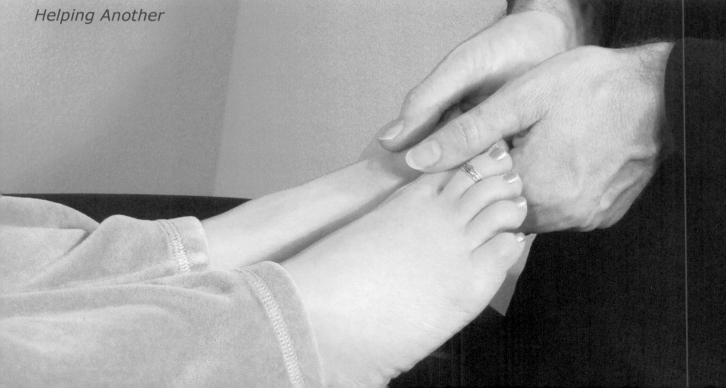

Holding base of skull and opposite collarbone

Compassionate Understanding may help connect you to your soul's desires, help clean your blood, and help bring every body-mind function into a general order.

This Quick Step may help with your eye "projects" too. And, in addition to all of that help, this *Healing Touch Quick Step* is another possible natural facelift helper.

Simply place your left hand on the left side back of your head at the base of your skull.

Place your right hand on your right collarbone.

Relax your shoulders, hands and fingers and exhale.

Breathe normally while holding your hands in this position for up to 5 minutes. It is that easy.

Then switch your hands and do the other side of the base of your skull and opposite side collarbone. Gently be with your body's natural system of healing for another 5 minutes.

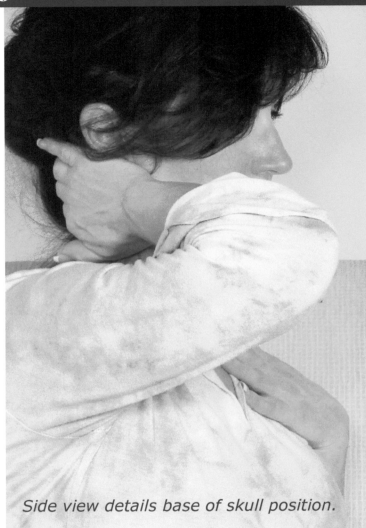

Side view details base of skull position.

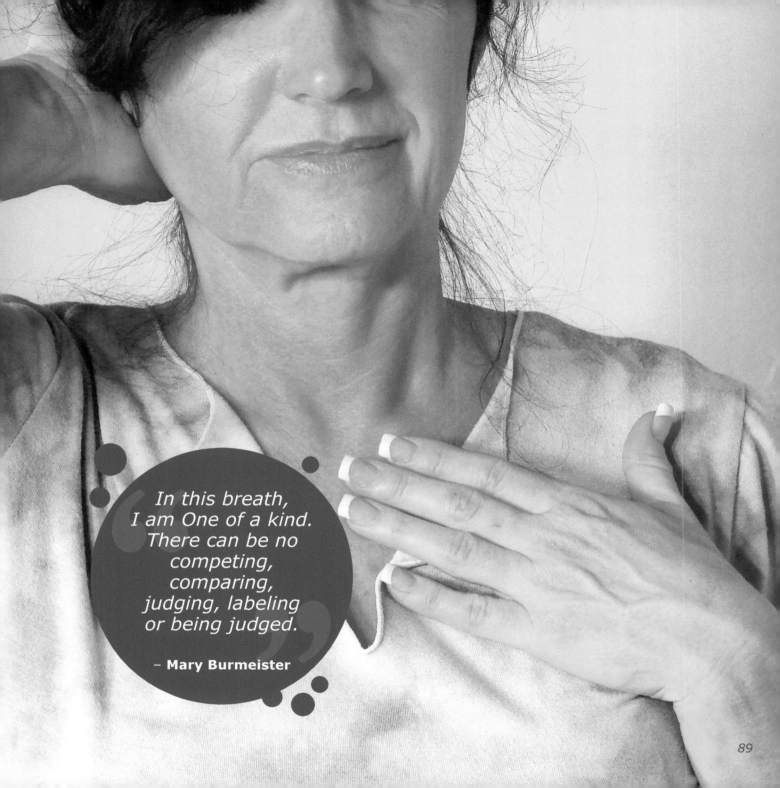

"In this breath,
I am One of a kind.
There can be no
competing,
comparing,
judging, labeling
or being judged.

– Mary Burmeister

Holding side of neck and opposite forehead

This *Healing Touch Quick Step* may be helpful for gall bladder "projects" because of the energy pathway flow pattern.

Decision Making Support may help with making decisions, as well as helping to harmonize over use of your eyes, and may help harmonize a headache.

Place your left hand on the left side of your neck.

Place your right hand on the right side forehead just above your eyebrow.

That is, side of your neck and your opposite forehead area.

Relax your shoulders, hands and fingers, and exhale.

Breathe normally and simply be with your body's natural healing system for up to 5 minutes.

Then switch your hand positions and do the other side of your head for up to 5 minutes.

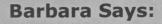

Barbara Says:

Once I heard Dorothy Maclean (Co-Founder of Findhorn, Scotland, 88 years young at the time) say that she tied a string around her finger to remind her to think of God every hour...

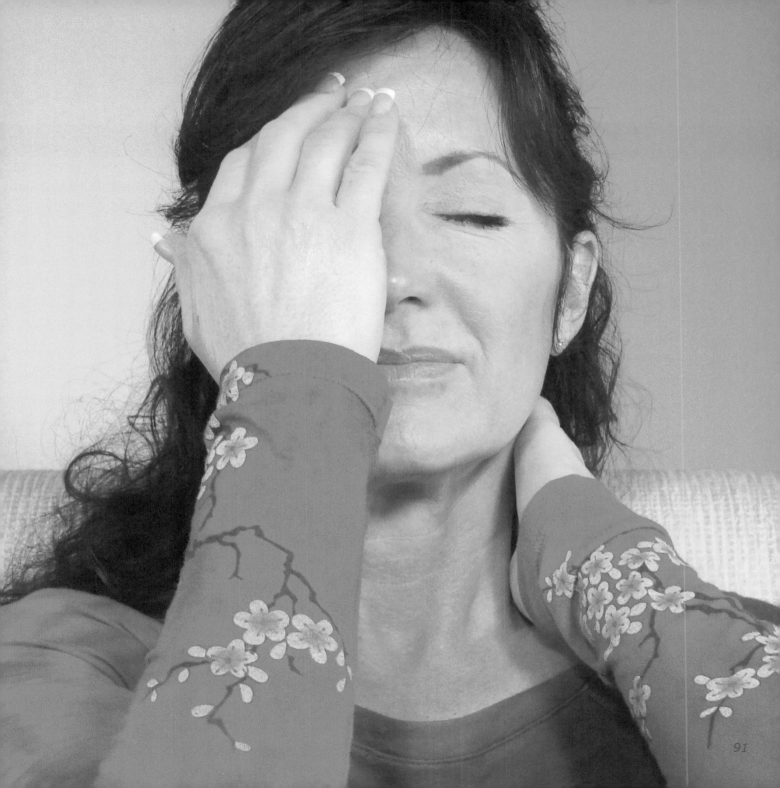

Holding front bottom rib and opposite elbow

Hot flashes? Cholesterol imbalances? This one may help.

Uplifts, Brings Vitality, Recharges Heart may be wonderful for anyone who works the night shift—nurses, doctors, gas station attendants, crew chiefs, soldiers.

How does it help? Because you are tapping into the body's natural, universal healing energy that flows through specific pathways that may address this need.

One very important possibility with this Quick Step is that it may help **cool the body**.

Place your left hand on the bottom of your right front ribcage.

Place your right hand on your left elbow at the elbow crease or the bend of elbow.

Relax your shoulders, hands and fingers, and exhale.

Breathe normally and gently be with your body's natural healing system for up to 5 minutes.

Then switch your hands to apply to the other side of your body for up to 5 minutes.

> " *Fatigue arises when you are not addressing the needs of the Soul.* "
>
> **–Manly P. Hall**

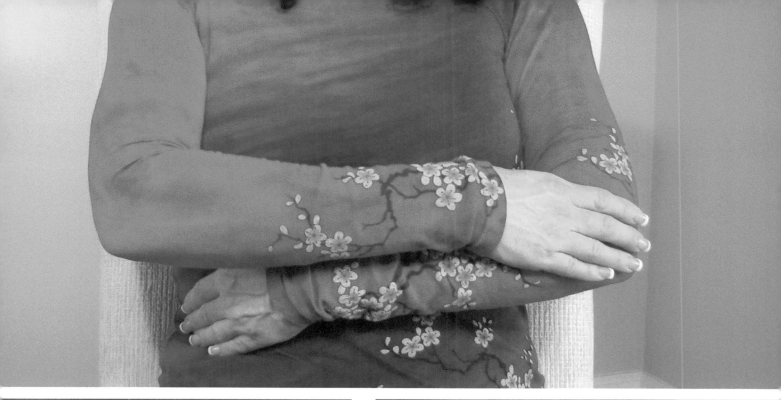

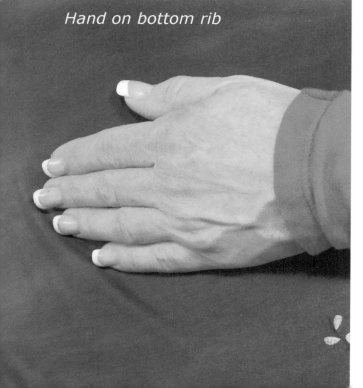

Hand on bottom rib

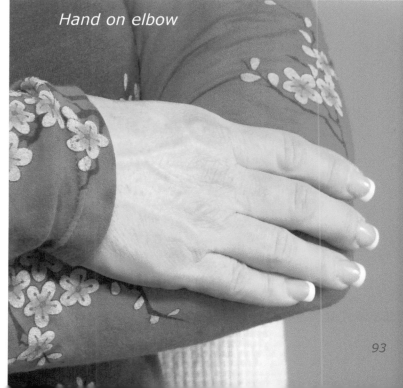

Hand on elbow

Elderly man's story with *Uplifts, Brings Vitality, Recharges Heart*

One late afternoon at the fitness center, I saw an elderly man stagger out of the sauna and almost fall into the Jacuzzi. Every part of his body that was visible— legs, arms, chest, face, head was an evenly bright red. He looked like someone had painted him fire engine red.

I happened to know the man and began engaging him in conversation to see if he was all right. His life force was so shallow that he spoke very faintly. He was not all right.

He was sitting in a chair near the pool and was acting agitated. He could not get comfortable. He put his head in his hands and bent over. Then he tried to cover his head with his towel and he put his head back down in his lap. He had been in a 179 degree extreme heat environment for 30 minutes or more, and he was a man in his 70's.

I asked if I could help him cool down his body. He said yes. I asked if I could place my hands on him. He said yes. First I gently touched his elbow, and placed my other hand on his opposite front rib so he could feel where to place his hands. I took a step back from him and applied the same *Healing Touch Quick Step* to myself so that he could see what I was doing.

The man mimicked what I was doing and placed his fingertips on his elbow and other hand on his opposite bottom rib. Within about 15 seconds (all the while he was talking softly about the delightful conversation he'd just had with an interesting fellow in the sauna) he said: "Oh my dear I am suddenly feeling better," exhaled and smiled.

He continued to hold his elbow and opposite bottom rib for maybe 5 minutes (I continued to hold mine too) and then I suggested "we" switch sides and do the other elbow and opposite rib for good measure. We did that.

I stayed with the man for about 10 minutes. Another woman in the pool and I continued to witness in amazement as the redness literally began to leave his body from the top of his face descending all the way down his face! One part of his face was now white, natural skin tone and there was a perfect horizontal dividing line across his face where the natural skin tone filled in and the red color was vanishing.

It seemed so surreal, as though his body was a bottle of red water and the red liquid was somehow effortlessly emptying itself out of this man's face and down the front of his body in a perfectly measured way, like the redness was being pulled out of his "container" from the bottoms of his feet.

His skin tone went from complete red to normal skin tone before our very eyes! The sound of his voice becoming stronger, and

Within about 15 seconds he said, "Oh my dear, I am suddenly feeling better!"

the man becoming more present also told me that his life force was coming out of its critical need. What happened to this man was very serious.

Heat exhaustion and heat stroke can cause organ failure and death. *Healing Touch Quick Steps* do not replace emergency medical care. The fitness center attendant, who was an emergency medical tech, came in to help.

And, by the time she had arrived, this man was markedly on the track of cooler health again. And I heard later that the man was back at the sauna every day after that, only this time for much less time. I thought to myself, he is acting as though nothing ever happened. I think I would have stayed out of the sauna for at least a few days. And, every person's harmony is different.

Holding elbow and opposite forehead

Here is a Quick Step that may be beneficial for infants, babies just for the goodness of it, and for "babies" of all ages too.

Protecting Your Organs may help someone who is in critical need. Respiratory, cardiovascular, blood chemistry, digestion, and elimination organ functions may be helped with this Quick Step.

One very important possibility with this Quick Step is that it may help **warm the body**, may help someone recovering from surgery or serious illness, as well as premature babies.

This one hand placement may help so much because in Eastern healing wisdom your body's natural system of healing pathways support all of these body functions.

Place your right hand on your left elbow at the elbow crease.

Place your left hand on your right forehead just above your eyebrow.

You can do this hand placement while resting your arms on a table or desk, and this Quick Step is also easily done while lying down.

Relax your shoulders, hands and fingers, and exhale.

Simply be with your body's natural healing system for up to 5 minutes.

Then switch hands to apply to the other side of your body for another 5 minutes.

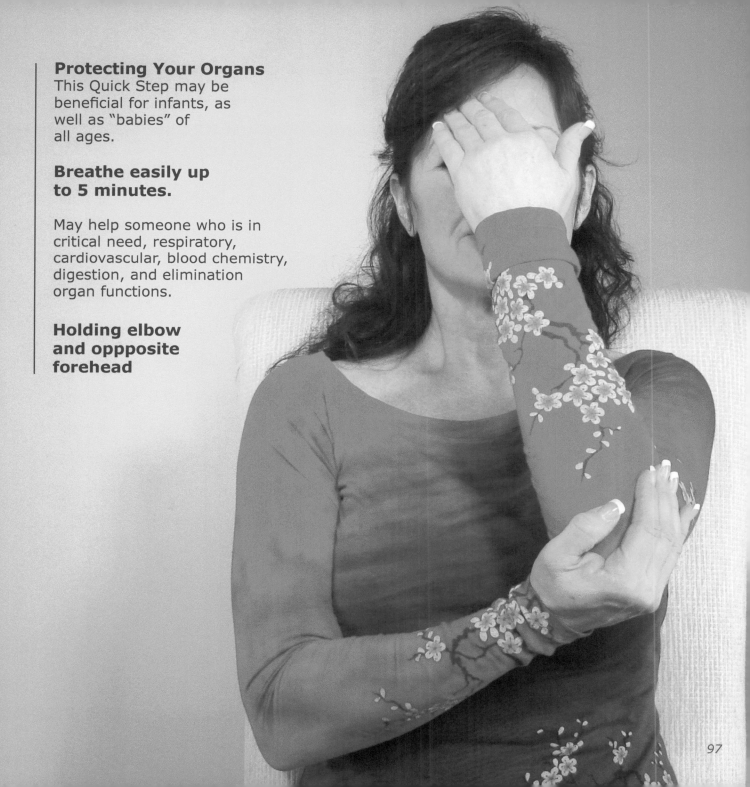

Protecting Your Organs
This Quick Step may be
beneficial for infants, as
well as "babies" of
all ages.

**Breathe easily up
to 5 minutes.**

May help someone who is in
critical need, respiratory,
cardiovascular, blood chemistry,
digestion, and elimination
organ functions.

**Holding elbow
and oppposite
forehead**

97

Holding shoulder and opposite breast area

Comfortable cholesterol, and flexible, healthy arteries may be supported here, and much more.

Take What You Need and Dump the Rest Quick Step self-care may help with elimination projects, and discernment, and may be very helpful for sore throats and fighting off a cold or flu.

Place your right hand on your right shoulder.

Place your left hand on your left breast/chest at the heart level.

Relax your shoulders, hands and fingers, and exhale.

Breathe normally and simply be with your body's natural healing system for up to 5 minutes.

Then switch your hand positions to apply to the other side of your body, relaxing and breathing normally while being with your body's natural healing system for an additional 5 minutes.

Barbara Says:

Remember, when you give yourself *Healing Touch Quick Steps* self-care, you are saying yes to your wholeness even if you are not sure what wholeness is.

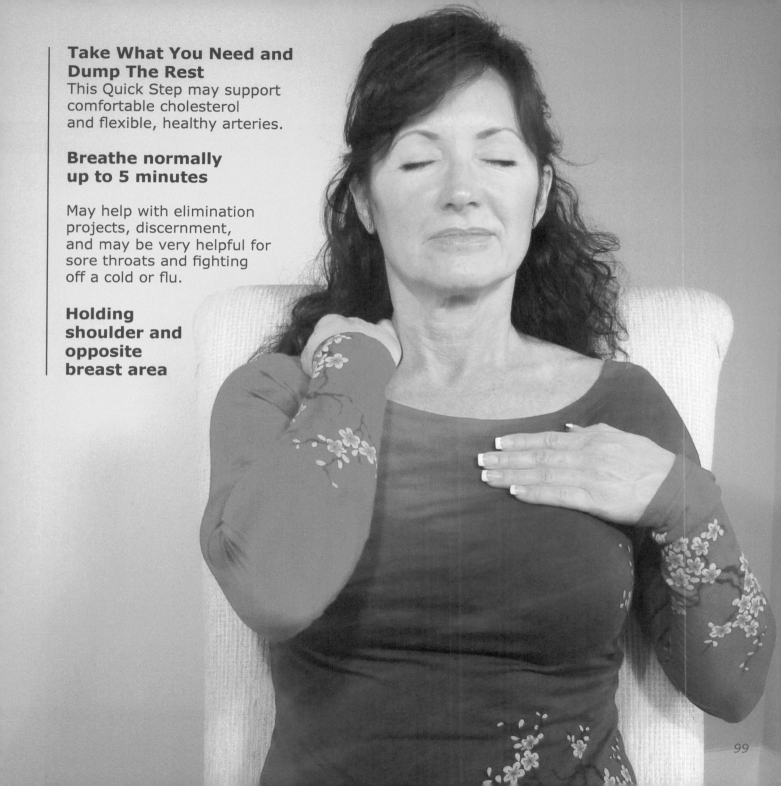

Take What You Need and Dump The Rest
This Quick Step may support comfortable cholesterol and flexible, healthy arteries.

Breathe normally up to 5 minutes

May help with elimination projects, discernment, and may be very helpful for sore throats and fighting off a cold or flu.

Holding shoulder and opposite breast area

Fingers in palms

If you want to help bring your past, present and your future all into peace and harmony, this may be the *Healing Touch Quick Step* for you.

Being With What Is may help connect you with your Big Picture Self and the Silence that holds all goodness, while helping to harmonize your breathing and heart rate, and calming the mind—a perfect 5-minute meditation.

Place the fingers of your right hand into the center of your left palm.

Place the fingers of your left hand into the center of the palm of your right hand.

Relax your shoulders, hands and fingers, and exhale.

Breathe normally and simply be with your body's natural healing system for up to 5 minutes.

Optional Position: You can either do fingertips in one hand at a time, as described above, OR you can rest your hands in your lap with the back of one hand in the palm of the other hand.

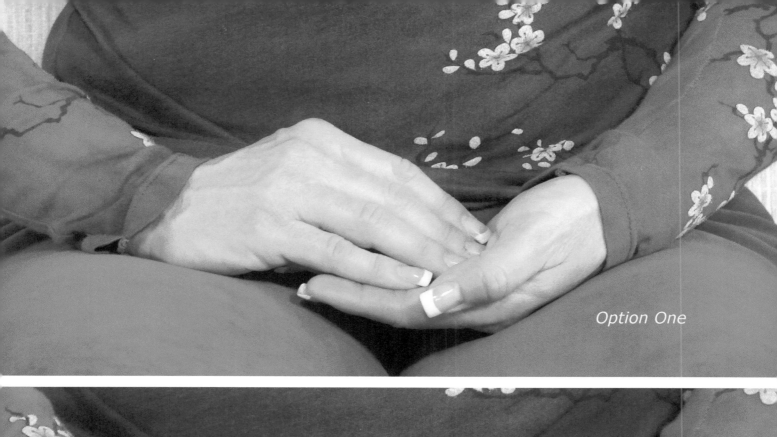

Option One

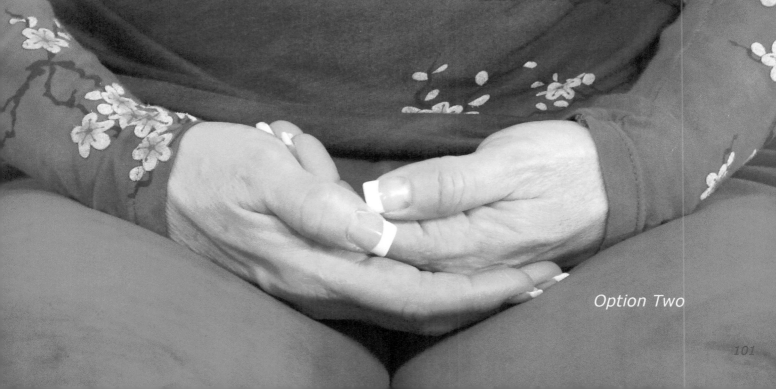

Option Two

Hands on sides with fingers on top of head

Have you ever felt really burnt out, totally spent and you don't have the energy for anything else?

This *Healing Touch Quick Step* called **Exhaustion Relief** may help you recover and revitalize your energy. This may also be very helpful for anyone who sits in front of a computer for long hours every day, as well as someone who is chronically fatigued.

First, place your hands on the sides of your head with your middle fingers touching at the top center of your head.

Then, slide your hands back down the sides of your head so that the base of each hand is resting just above the tops of your ears.

That's it! How simple is this?

Relax your shoulders, and exhale.

Breathe normally and simply be with your body's natural system of healing for up to 5 minutes.

If your arms get tired, you can do this one easily while lying down and resting your arms on a pillow.

If a behavior by you or someone in your life does not nurture and support your thriving, best self, let it go.

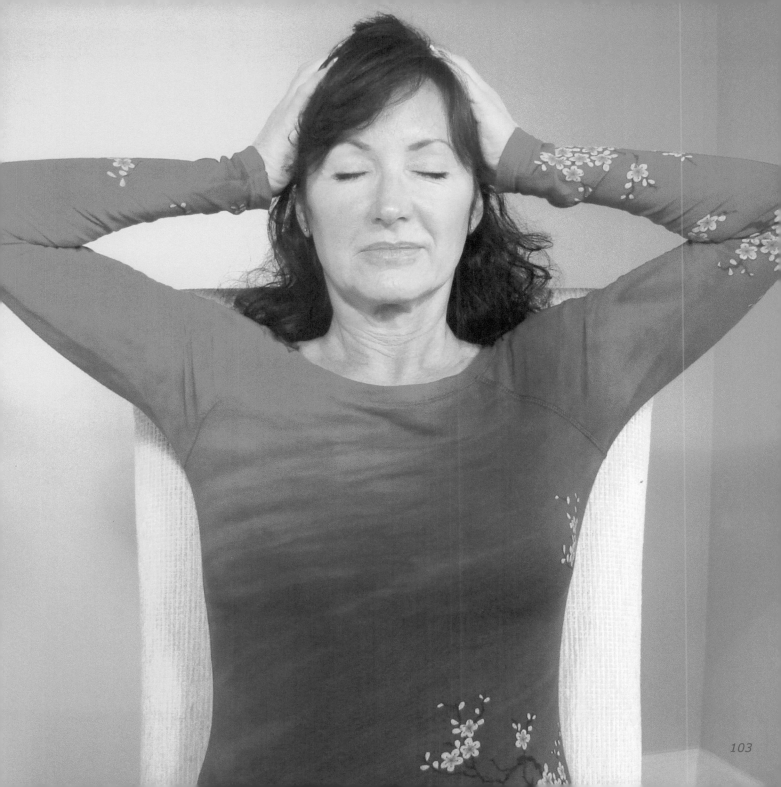

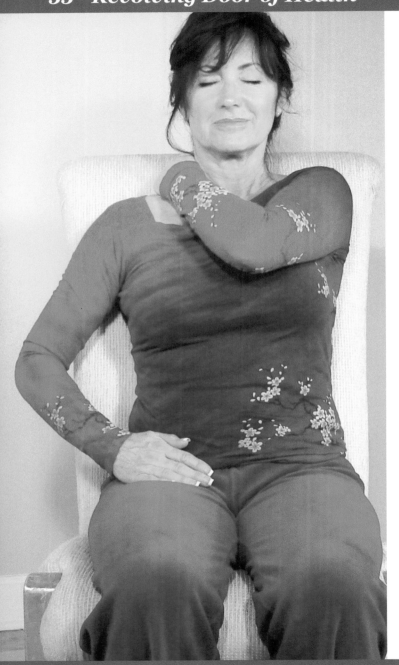

Hand on shoulder with fingers pointing to spine and same side groin area

This one may possibly promote a natural antibiotic activity.

This *Healing Touch Quick Step* gives you a visual image of a revolving or swinging door. Some Eastern energy philosophies suggest a healthy immune system should push out an invader bug in the half breath (or nano-second) that it is noticed by the body, like a swinging door that pushes it right back out of the system.

This is the idea behind **Revolving Door of Health** *Healing Touch Quick Step*—a built-in, fast acting, graceful defense mechanism.

Revolving Door of Health may help harmonize fever, cold or flu, in addition to whatever other remedies you are using to defend your body.

This may be specific help because you are tapping into your body's natural healing system that addresses the energy pathways for these particular needs.

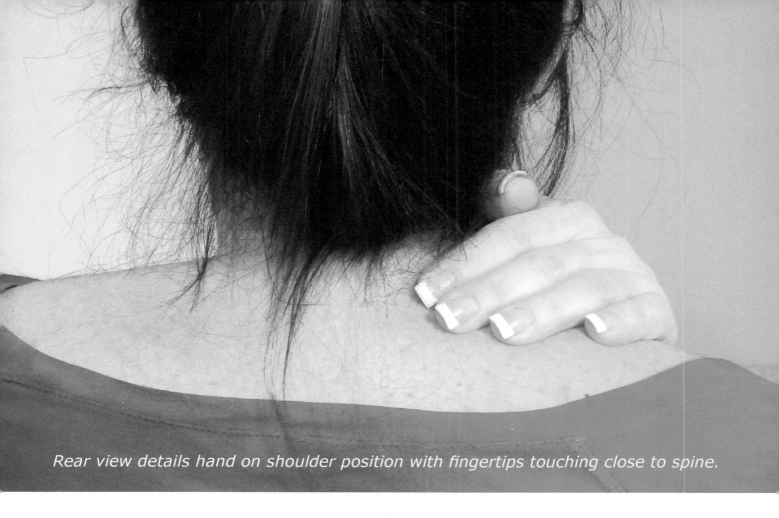

Rear view details hand on shoulder position with fingertips touching close to spine.

Place your left hand on your right shoulder with your fingertips resting on the top of the right side of your back to the outside of your spine.

Place your right hand on the right groin area at the place where your leg meets your torso.

Relax your shoulders, hands and fingers, and exhale.

Simply be with your body's natural healing system for up to 5 minutes.

If you have time, apply the Quick Step to the other side of your body.

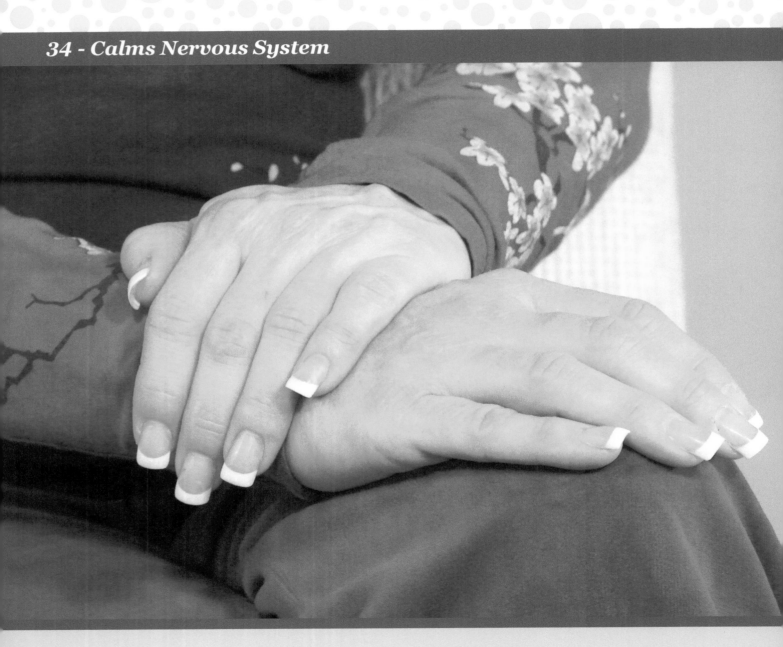

Holding outside of wrist (little finger side of wrist)

Calms Nervous System may help with motion sickness, nausea, and shaky head or limbs, and may also help if you are nervous for a big job interview or speaking in front of a crowd and no one will even know you are helping your Self.

Place your left hand on the little finger side of your right hand at the wrist.

Relax your shoulders, hands and fingers and exhale.

Breathe normally while holding the little finger side of your wrist for up to 5 minutes.

Be sure to apply your self-care Quick Step to your other wrist for another 5 minutes.

With *Healing Touch Quick Steps* energy healing self help, over time it may be possible to interrupt chronic conditions forever.

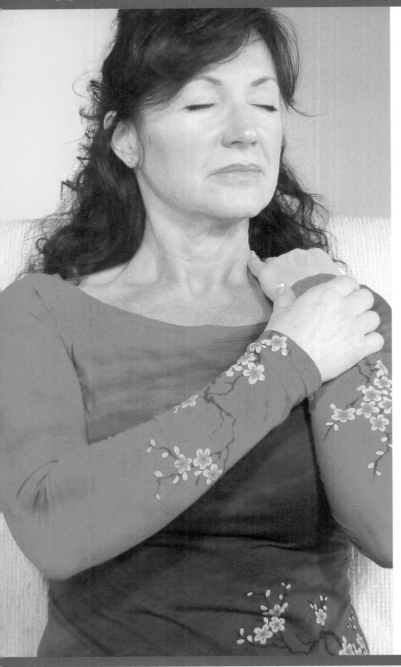

Shoulder and same side outer wrist

Heart Wholeness may help anything to do with the heart – emotional and physical, and may help arteries, blood vessels, and circulation.

Heart Wholeness may be a good first choice for helping harmonize heart functions because you are tapping into your body's natural system of healing of specific energy pathways that flow through these areas.

Consider thinking about flexibility of your arteries.

Place your left hand on your left shoulder.

Place your right hand on your left wrist at the **little finger side** of your wrist.

Relax your shoulders, hands and fingers, and exhale.

Breathe normally and simply be with your body's natural healing system for up to 5 minutes.

Then switch hand positions for an additional 5 minutes.

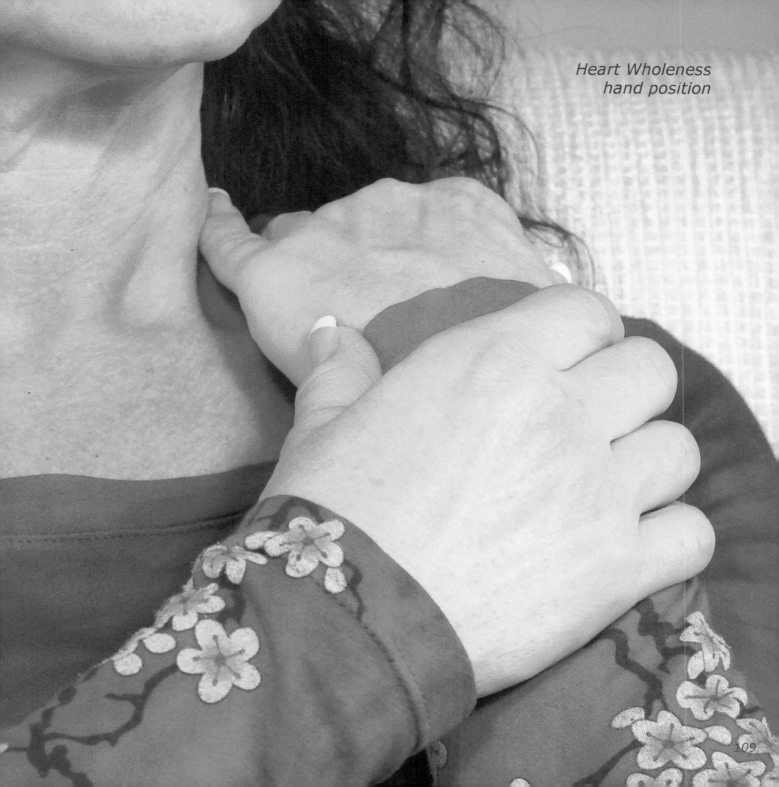

Heart Wholeness
hand position

109

Finger Harmonizers

You may experience significant emotional balancing help by holding each of your fingers. You can rest your hands in your lap for the finger holding Quick Steps.

The colors on this lovely hand represent colors of harmony for each of the emotions that may be harmonized by holding a particular finger.

On an energetic level, when your emotions are harmonized, there is no thing going on except clear space and the breath.

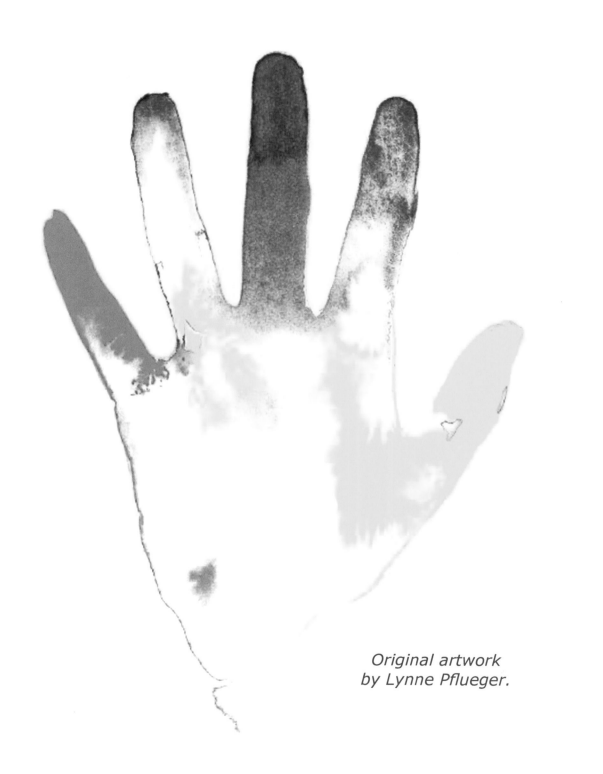

Original artwork by Lynne Pflueger.

36 - Harmonizing Worry

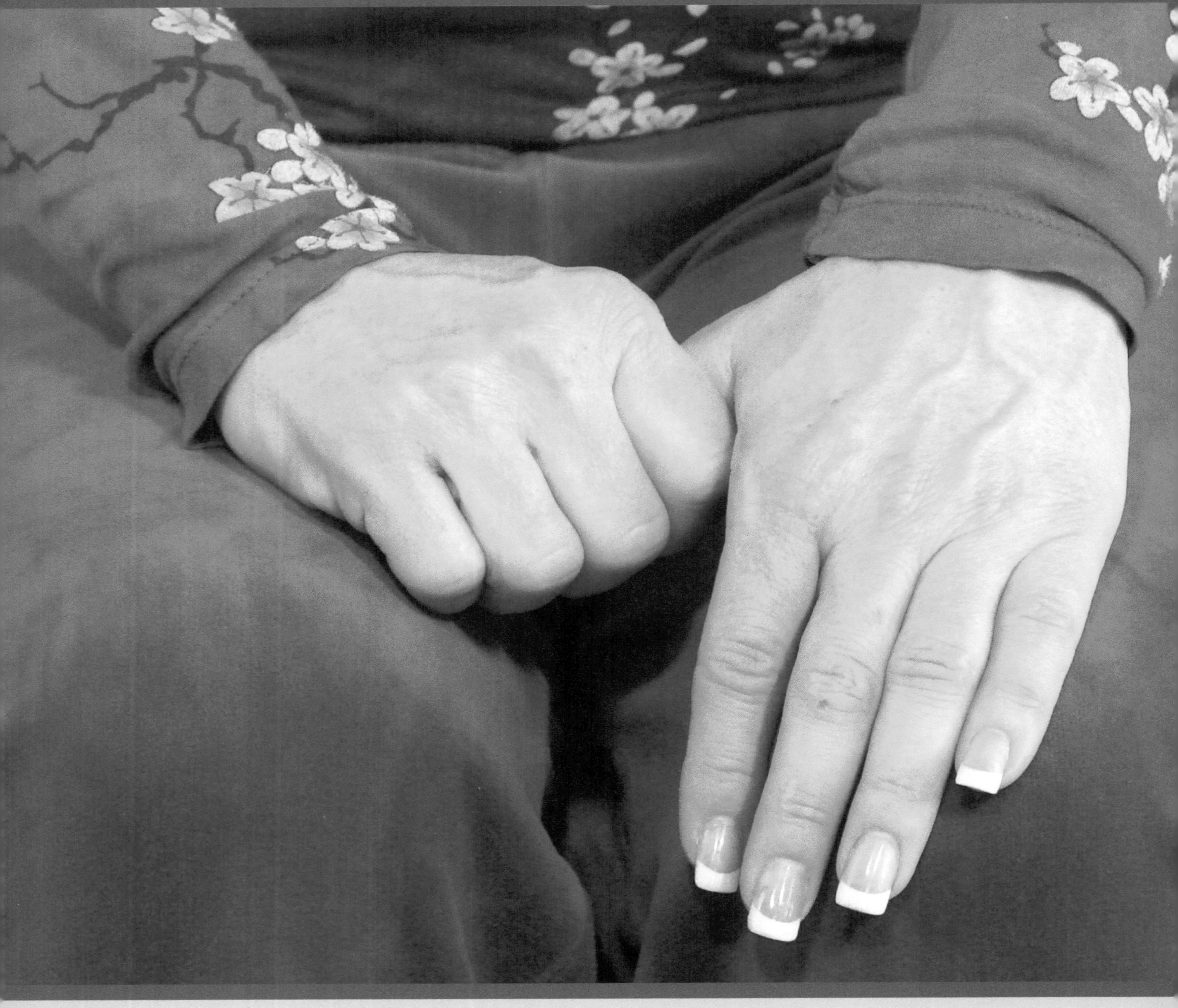

Holding the thumb

Harmonizing Worry Quick Step may help what it says—worry. It may also be helpful for digestion functions, communication projects, healthy boundaries of all kinds, as well as unity and oneness consciousness. Oriental Medicine says that when you worry, your pulsing energy may feel stagnate, gummy and muddy.

Harmonizing Worry may ease you out of your head and get things moving.

Simply wrap your thumb and fingers of your right hand around your left THUMB. You may help harmonize worry and get your energy happily and healthily flowing again.

Relax your shoulders, hands and fingers, and exhale.

Breathe normally and simply be with your body's natural healing system for up to 5 minutes.

Then switch your hand position and do the same to your other thumb for another 5 minutes.

J's story about harmonizing with the fingers

"I have been using your Healing Touch Quick Steps every day. Mostly I've been doing those that allow deep relaxation and the ones that use 'holding of the fingers.' They are having the desired effect, and I am able to rest more deeply, for which I am most grateful."

–J

Louise's story about emotional help with the finger harmonizers

"I LOVE these healing quick steps! I feel so grateful to have this resource. That it is immediate and easy, and that you can do it in the flow of life - whatever is going on – is so precious.

"I was watching a documentary that I knew would bring up my anger for me. I did the Quick Step for anger while watching the film and I was able to stay clear and present in observation rather than become emotionally upset."

–Louise Deerfield

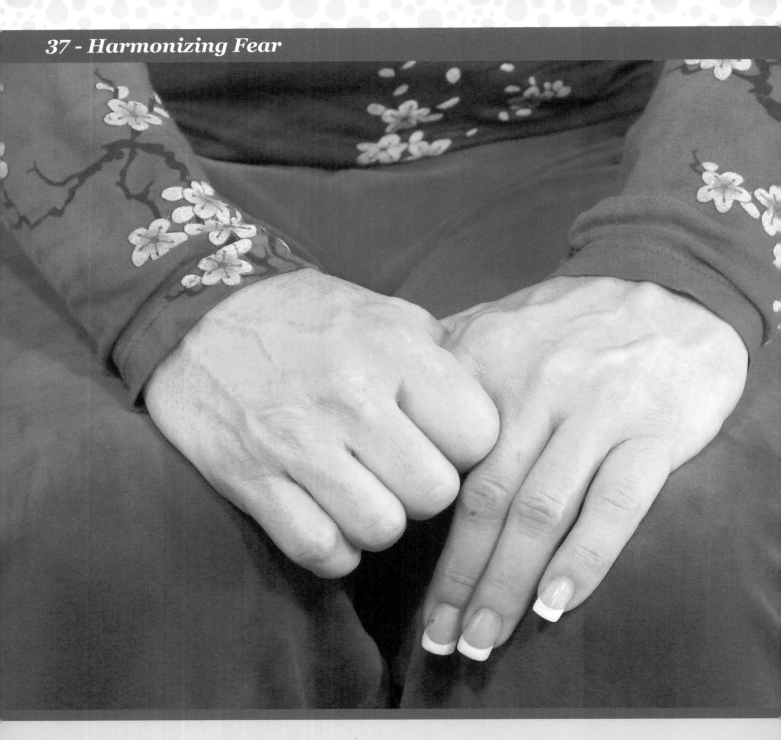

Holding the index finger

Harmonizing Fear Quick Step may help harmonize, you guessed it - fear. It may also help harmonize elimination discomforts and your natural flow of energy.

Harmonizing your emotions may help everything in your life go more smoothly. When you are standing in fear, your energy descends and cannot rise. When fear is harmonized, you may be able to relax and receive nourishing, energizing life force to live your life well.

Simply wrap your thumb and fingers of your right hand around your left INDEX finger.

Relax your shoulders, hands and fingers, and exhale.

Breathe normally and simply be with your body's natural healing system for up to 5 minutes.

Then switch your hand position and hold your other index finger for another 5 minutes.

Harmonizing Fear. Easy does it.

> " *The kingdom of God does not come in such a way as to be seen. No one will say, 'Look, here it is!' or 'There it is!' because the kingdom of God is within you.* "

–Luke
New Testament

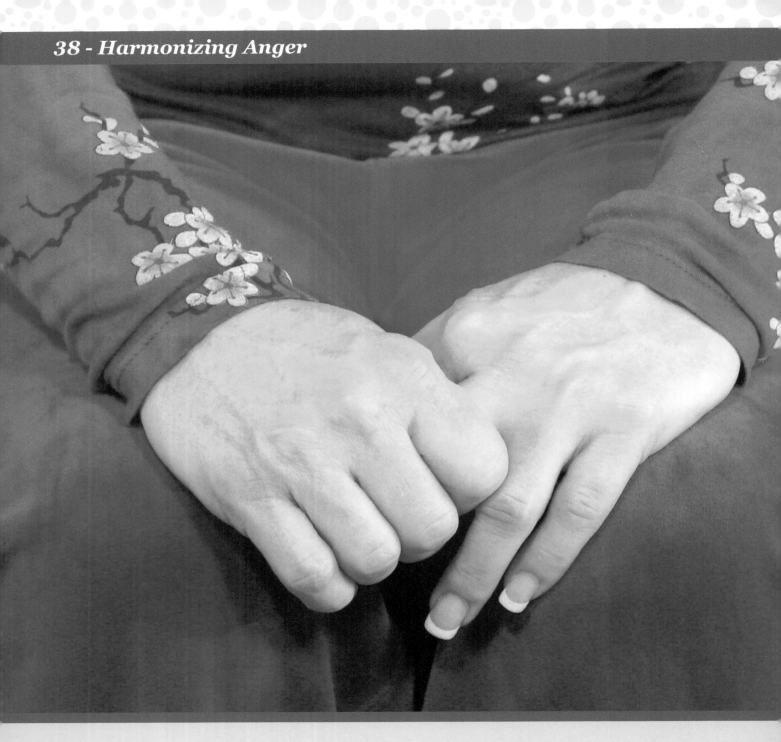

Holding the middle finger

Yes, the middle finger.

Harmonizing Anger may help harmonize anger. It may also help harmonize compassionate understanding as well as anything in the vertical center of the body, from head to toes, toes to head, and everything in between because in terms of energy relationships, the middle finger relates to the middle, vertical center of your body.

When you are feeling angry, your life force energy rises hot and fast.

Applying **Harmonizing Anger** Quick Step self-care may help initiate a cooling down, breathing away negativity, and help you come into common sense and an easing away the anger.

Wrap your thumb and fingers of your right hand around your left MIDDLE finger.

Relax your shoulders, hands and fingers, and exhale.

Breathe normally and simply be present with your body's natural healing system for up to 5 minutes.

Then switch hands and hold your other middle finger for 5 minutes.

Is whatever you are doing in the moment strengthening or weakening your Life Force flow?

Harmonizing Anger. Easy does it.

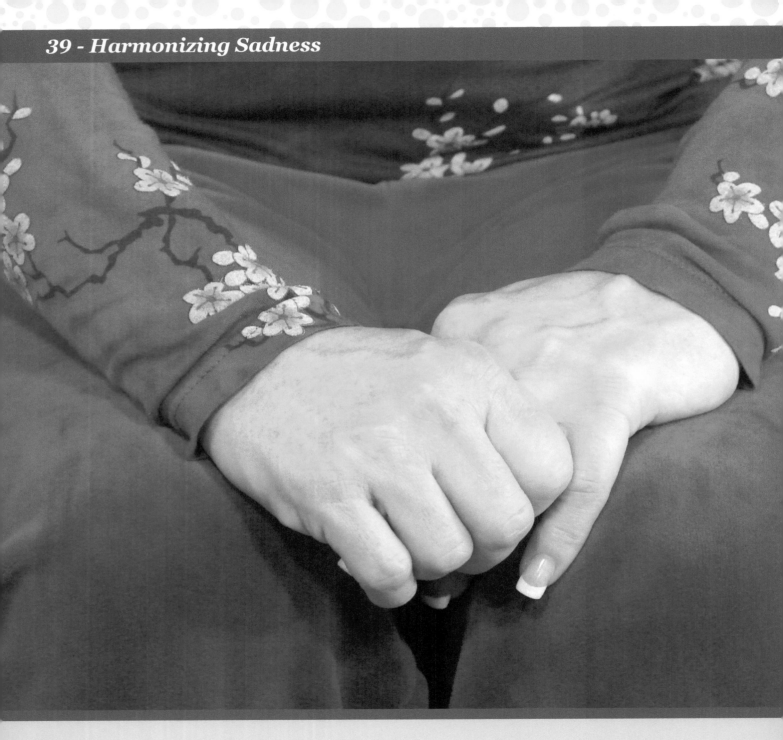

Holding the ring finger

Harmonizing Sadness Quick Step may help harmonize sadness and grief as well as breathing and lung functions.

When you grieve and experience sadness, your energy disperses, depletes.

Harmonizing Sadness Quick Step may help gently rebuild your energy, and give you strength and courage to live your life well.

Wrap your thumb and finger of your right hand around your left RING finger to help harmonize sadness and grief.

Relax your shoulders, hands and fingers, and exhale.

Breathe normally and simply be with your body's natural healing system for up to 5 minutes.

Then switch hands and hold your other ring finger for 5 minutes.

Harmonizing Sadness. Easy does it.

> *What the caterpillar calls the end of the world, the master calls the butterfly.*
>
> **—Mary Burmeister**

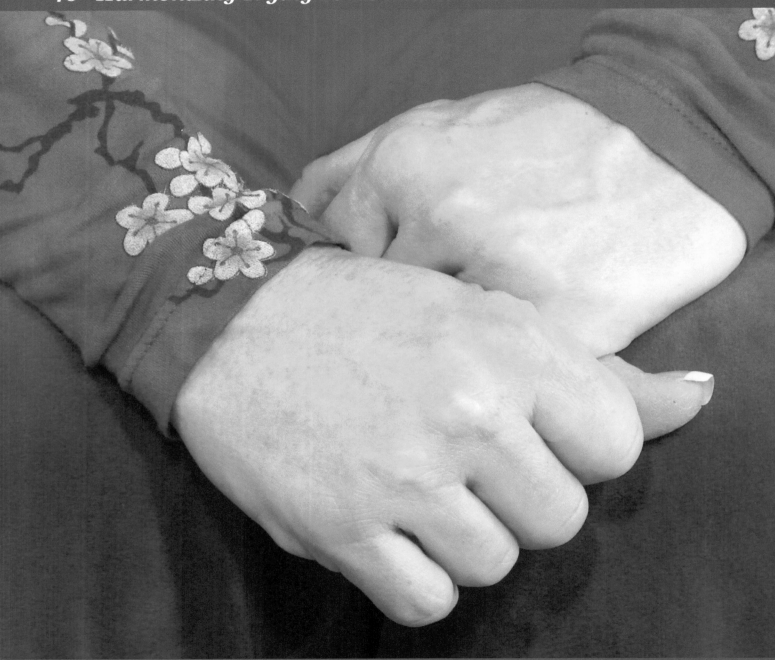

Holding the little finger

Harmonizing Trying to Do and Be Too Much Quick Step may help harmonize feeling anxious or scattered, laughing on the outside, crying on the inside, pretending or feigning or making believe one is something or someone one is not, shoulder tensions or disturbances and especially trying to do this or that or be this or that.

When you are trying to do this and trying to do that, being who you think you "should" be rather than who you are, your energy can get too fired up and scatter causing anxiety and a sense of feeling scattered.

So **Harmonizing Trying to Do and Be Too Much** Quick Step may help you ease into calm and centeredness and a sense of wholeness.

Wrap your thumb and fingers of your right hand around your left LITTLE finger.

Relax your shoulders, hands and fingers, and exhale.

Rest your hands in your lap while you apply this Quick Step self-care.

Breathe normally and simply be with your body's natural healing system for up to 5 minutes.

Then switch hands and hold your other little finger for another 5 minutes.

Self help cannot be overdone, unless it becomes obsessive.

Harmonizing Trying to Do and Be Too Much. Easy does it.

There are 5 steps to this Quick Step. Holding a finger and an opposite toe: Hold each finger-toe connection for 1 to 2 minutes.

This one is best given to you by someone else. **Magnificent Circulation** Quick Step is outstanding for anyone recovering from surgery of any kind, as well as all kinds of pain, or who is in the hospital or bedridden. This *Healing Touch Quick Step* may help reconnect the energy of any place that has been cut.

You will find it easier and more comfortable to hold a finger and an opposite toe while sitting or standing at the person's side near the person's ankles.

With this Quick Step you are making a diagonal connection with a hand and opposite foot. The energy connection is one finger and an opposite toe. Hold on to as much of the finger and the toe as you can.

As the giver of this energy healing help, be sure YOUR shoulders, arms and hands, your back and body positioning are as relaxed as possible.

Receiver, you relax and simply receive.

Step One:
THUMB and opposite LITTLE TOE

Step Two:
INDEX FINGER and opposite RING TOE.

Step Three:
MIDDLE FINGER and the opposite MIDDLE TOE.

Step Four:
RING FINGER and opposite INDEX TOE.

Step Five:
LITTLE FINGER and the opposite BIG TOE.

THEN switch sides of your friend's body, sitting or standing near her ankle and complete the other diagonal connection.

Magnificent Circulation Quick Step may also be helpful **for your pets too**.

Simply hold a front paw and an opposite back paw or as close to the paws as possible.

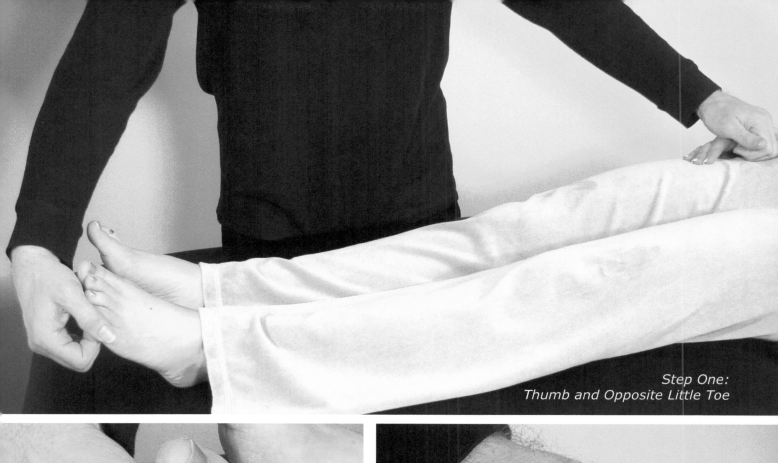

Step One:
Thumb and Opposite Little Toe

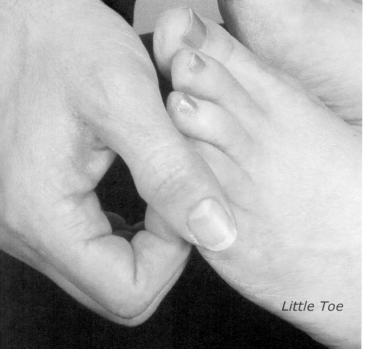

Little Toe

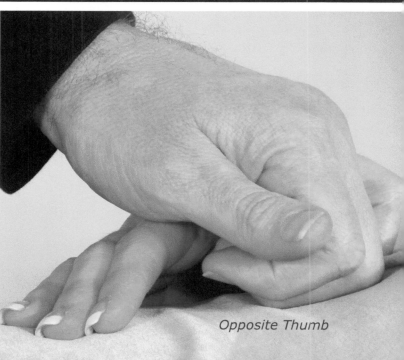

Opposite Thumb

Vesta's story with *Magnificent Circulation*

"During our 20 minute healing, I noticed immediately that energy was going to the area of the incisions. I felt calmer and more optimistic.

I feel sure that the **Magnificent Circulation** *Healing Touch Quick Step Barbara gave me to do on myself and have my sister help me with had a positive influence on my recovery from surgery."*

– Vesta Armstrong
Attorney at Law

...*this Quick Step had a positive influence on my recovery from surgery.*

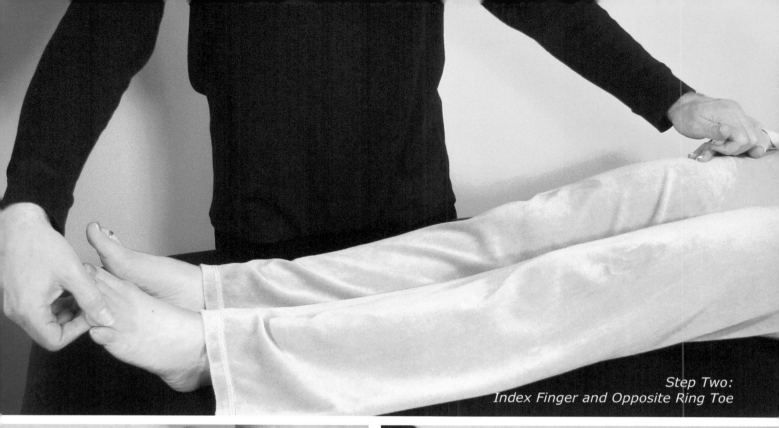

Step Two:
Index Finger and Opposite Ring Toe

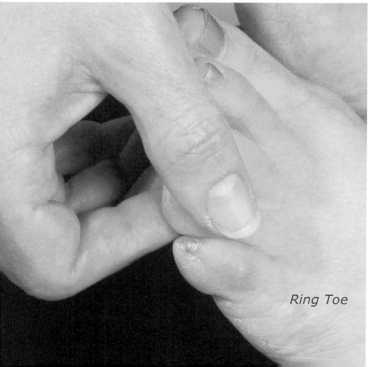

Ring Toe

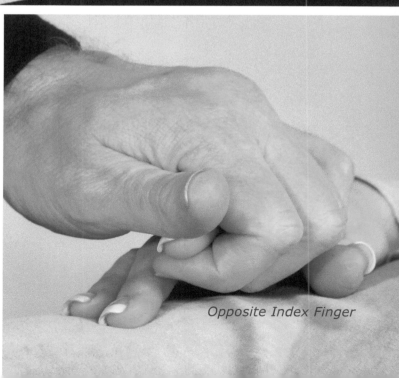

Opposite Index Finger

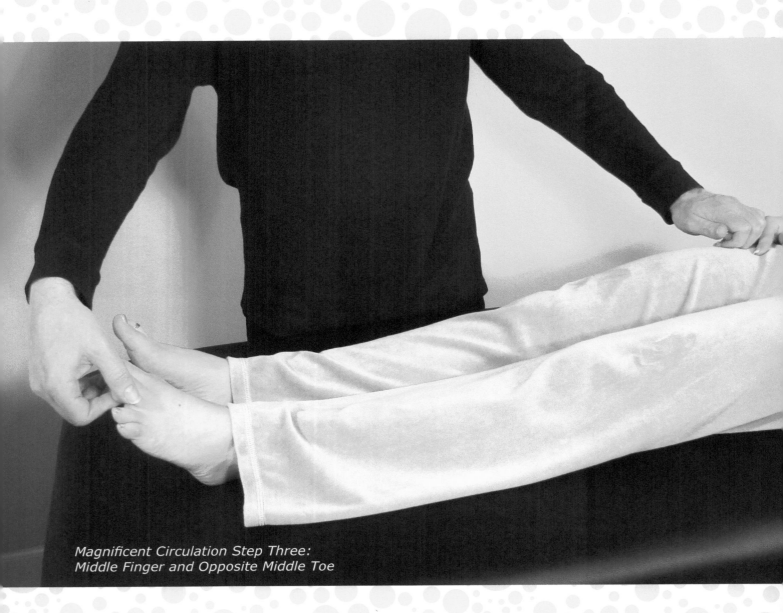

Magnificent Circulation Step Three:
Middle Finger and Opposite Middle Toe

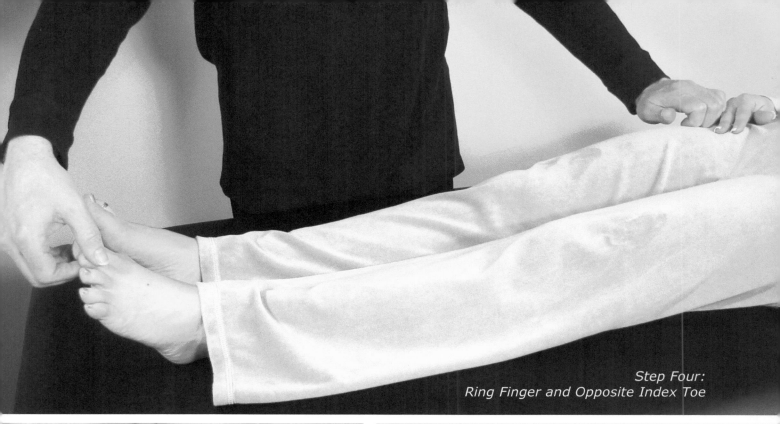

Step Four:
Ring Finger and Opposite Index Toe

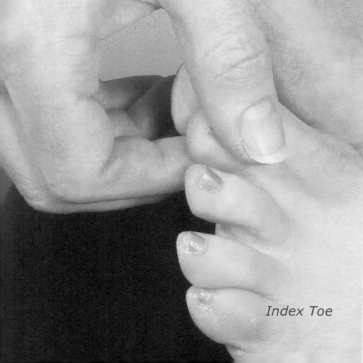

Index Toe

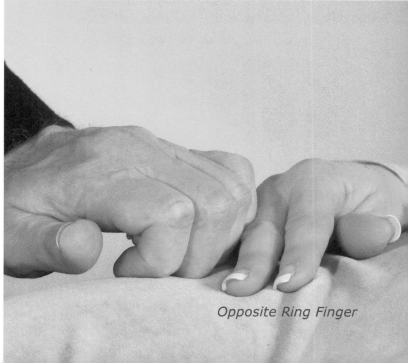

Opposite Ring Finger

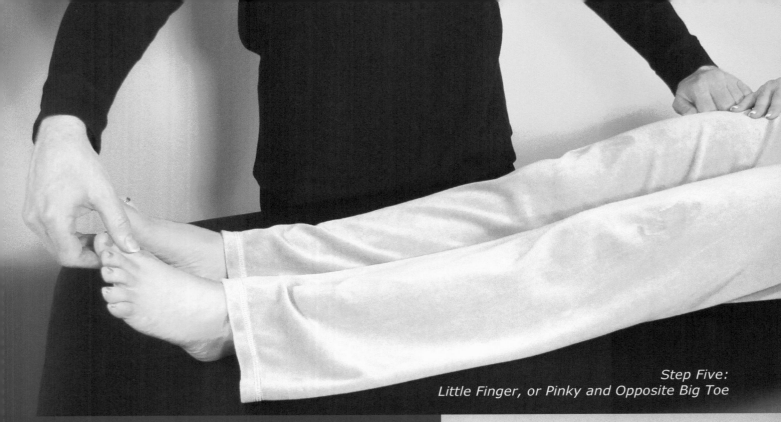

Step Five:
Little Finger, or Pinky and Opposite Big Toe

Quick Steps in Action

Larry's story with *Magnificent Circulation*

> " *I was wearing my steel reinforced toe work boots. She had one hand on the boot, other hand on my opposite hand. I felt the pain in my knee and hip release almost immediately. I felt circulation in both of my toes for the first time in 2 years!* "

–Larry
Construction Worker

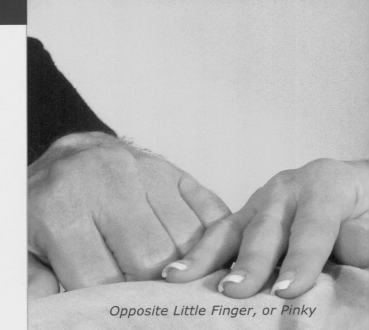

Opposite Little Finger, or Pinky

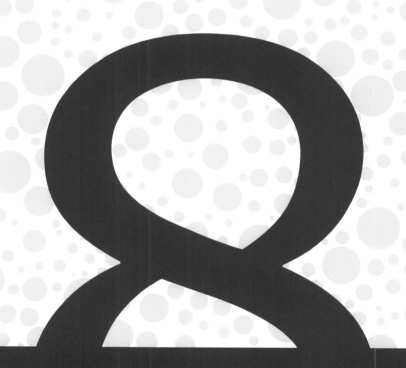

8 Really Fun "1-Step Helpers" Begin Here

Collarbone and same side bottom front rib

Happy Lungs may be helpful for breathing and respiratory concerns, asthma, common sense, immaturity, balancing body, mind and spirit, and may be helpful for mothers-to-be in the 6th and 8th months of pregnancy.

Place your right hand on your left collarbone.

Place your left hand on your left bottom front rib.

Relax your shoulders, arms and hands and simply be with your body's natural system of healing for up to 5 minutes.

Then switch sides and do the other side of your body, same side collarbone and same side bottom front rib for the same amount of time.

> " [S]he who knows others is wise. [S]he who knows herself is enlightened.
>
> **- Tao Te Ching** *(600 BCE)* "

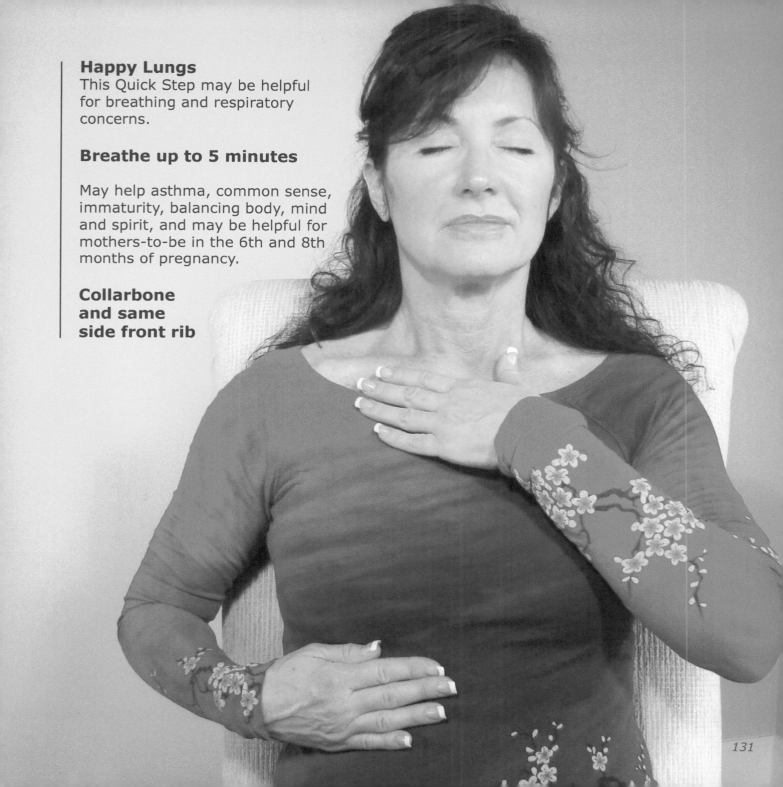

Happy Lungs
This Quick Step may be helpful for breathing and respiratory concerns.

Breathe up to 5 minutes

May help asthma, common sense, immaturity, balancing body, mind and spirit, and may be helpful for mothers-to-be in the 6th and 8th months of pregnancy.

Collarbone and same side front rib

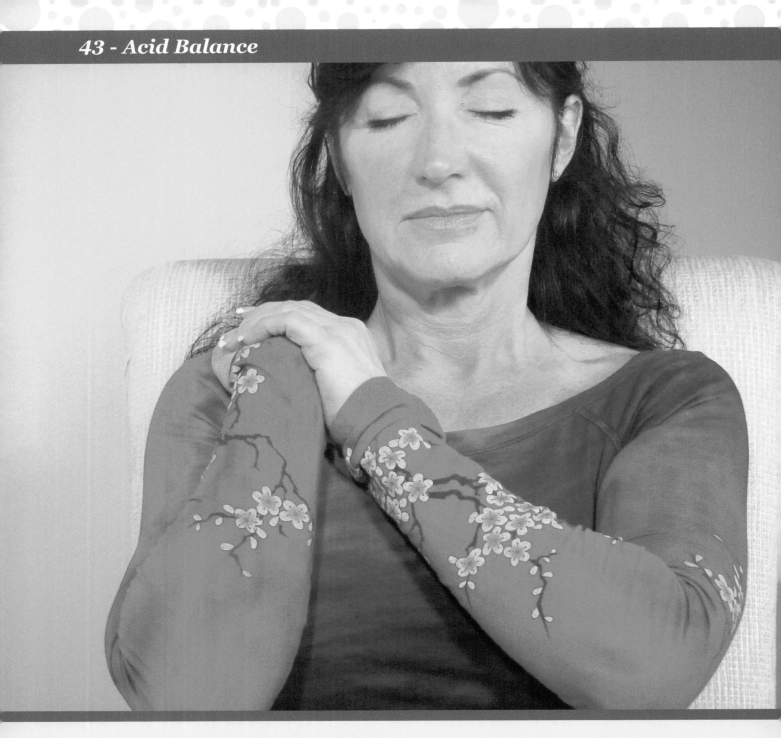

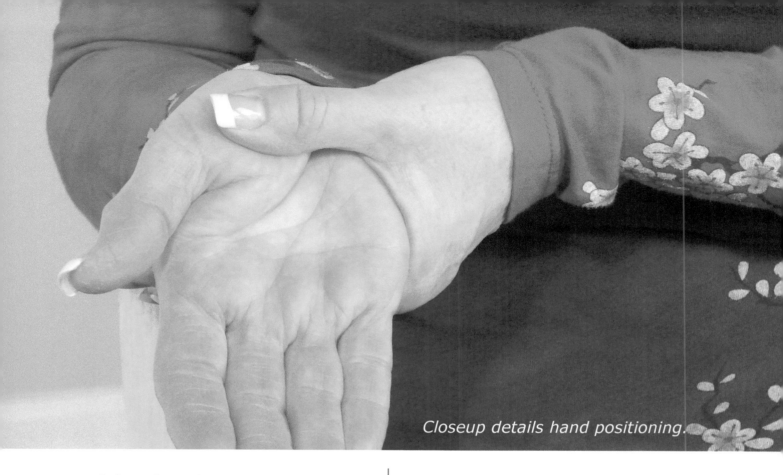

Closeup details hand positioning.

Base of thumb and same side shoulder

This Quick Step may be helpful for insomnia, releasing the pain of the past and anxiousness of tomorrow, and the pH of the body.

Place one hand on the base of your thumb and **then place** the hand you are holding on that same side shoulder.

Relax your shoulders, arms and hands as much as possible.

Exhale and simply be with your body's natural system of healing for up to 5 minutes.

Then switch sides and do the other side for the same amount of time.

Little toe and outside of same side ankle

This *Healing Touch Quick Step* may be very valuable immediately after a stroke, has been considered a good general preventive Quick Step, and may be helpful for reducing scar tissue.

Very simply, **bend your right leg** and rest it on your left leg.

With your left hand "cradle" your ankle with your fingers touching the outside of the ankle.

With your right hand, hold your little toe.

Relax your shoulders, arms and hands as much as possible and simply be with your body's natural system of healing for up to 5 minutes.

Then switch and do the other side.

Note:
You may also administer this Quick Step to help someone else.

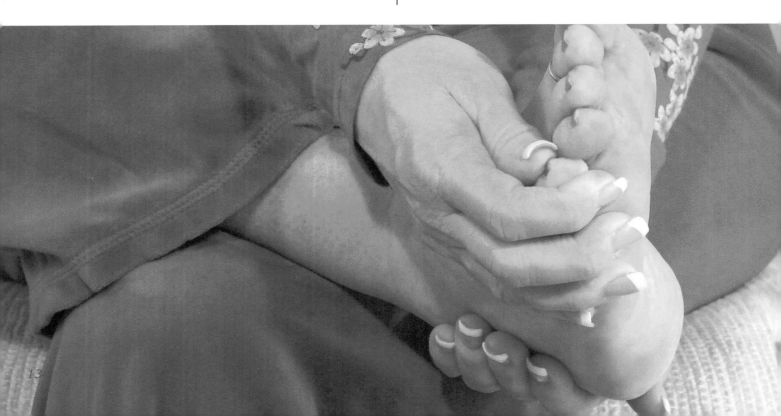

Helping Another

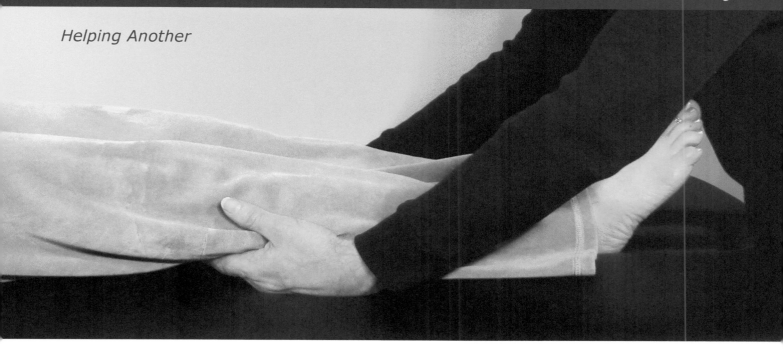

Palming the calves

This Quick Step may be helpful for severe burns, sunburn, teenage acne, and hot flashes.

If applied every day for 2 weeks may be a natural facelift.

When helping someone else simply place your flat palms fingertips as shown above on the back of both calves.

Relax your shoulders, arms and hands, exhale and simply be with your body's natural system of healing for up to 5 minutes.

Note:
You may also administer this Quick Step to yourself by placing your palms, fingers pointed down, on your calves.

Arch of foot and little toe

This *Healing Touch Quick Step* may be helpful for pains that move around the body.

Bend your right leg and rest it on your left leg.

Hold little toe with your left hand and **place your right hand** on the inside arch of your foot.

Relax your shoulders, arms, hands and fingers.

Exhale and simply be with your body's natural system of healing for up to 5 minutes.

Then switch and do the other foot.

Note:
You may also administer this Quick Step to help someone else *(see lower photo opposite page)*.

Deep inner peace is just a thought/feeling away. To experience peace does not mean that your life is always blissful. It means you are capable of tapping into a blissful state of mind amidst the normal chaos of a hectic life.

–Jill Bolte Taylor, Ph.D., *My Stroke of Insight*

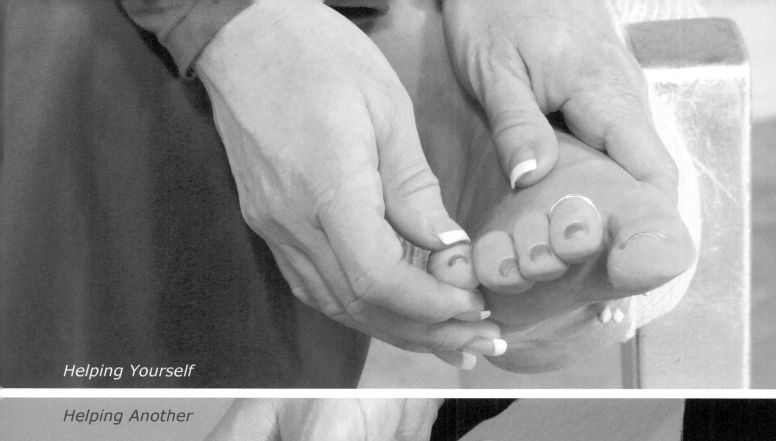
Helping Yourself

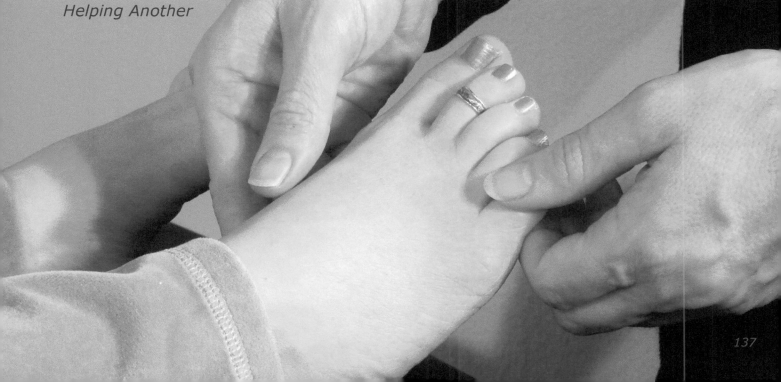
Helping Another

Inside and outside of ankle

Personal Analgesic may help harmonize ankles, bones, and feelings of panic as well as pain.

Hold the inside and outside of your ankle making sure your right hand is always on the inside of your ankle.

Relax your shoulders, arms, hands and fingers.

Exhale and simply be with your body's natural system of healing for up to 5 minutes.

Then switch feet and hold for the same amount of time.

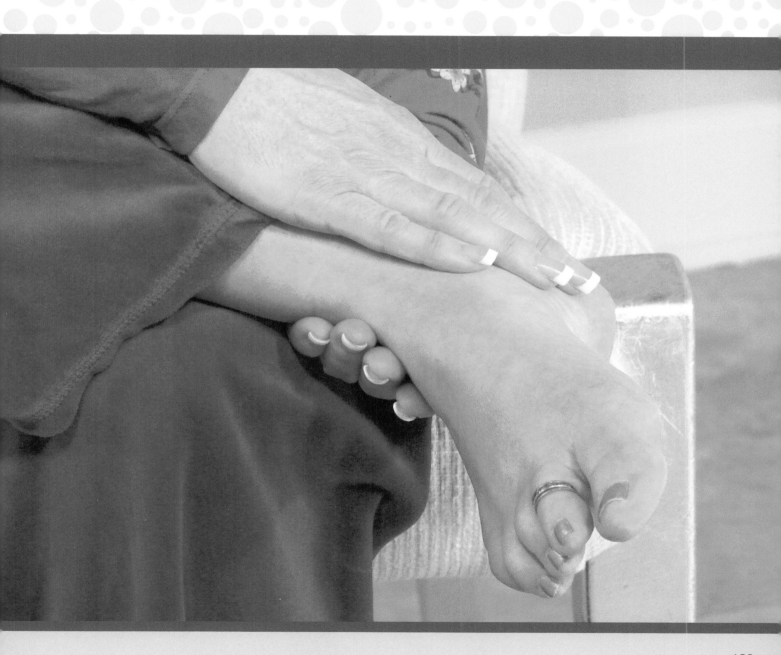

Groin and same side back of hip

This Quick Step may be very helpful for bronchial and respiratory needs, as well as grief, and of course phlegm clearing. When a person is feeling "under the weather," this one may be very comforting to give them.

When applying to another, place one flat hand gently at groin area as shown.

Place your other flat hand on the same side back of hip just below the waist.

Relax your shoulders, arms, hands, and exhale.

Simply be with your body's natural system of healing for up to 5 minutes.

Then switch and do the other side groin area and same side back of hip.

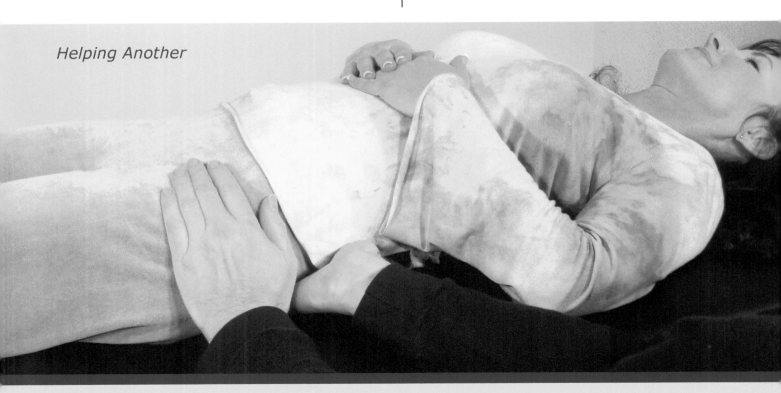

Helping Another

Shoulder and same side elbow crease.

Bones Help may help harmonize skeletal projects, bones, calcifications and lubrication of all of the joints.

Bend your left arm and **place** your left hand on your left shoulder.

Now place your right fingertips into the bend of your left elbow.

That's it!

Relax your shoulders, arms, hands, fingers, and exhale.

Simply be with your body's natural system of healing for up to 5 minutes.

Then switch sides and do the other shoulder and same side elbow crease for the same amount of time.

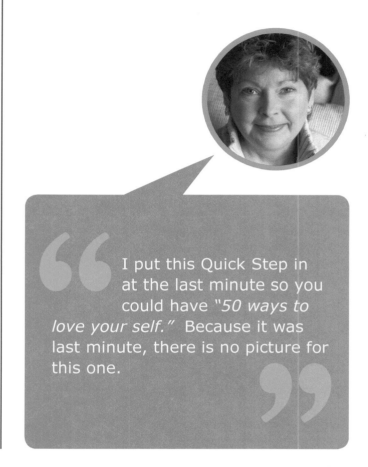

"I put this Quick Step in at the last minute so you could have *"50 ways to love your self."* Because it was last minute, there is no picture for this one."

Combining Quick Steps for Specific Health Projects

You may decide you want extra healing beyond your 3- to 5-minute experience.

For a particular health project, I suggest combining a few of the *Healing Touch Quick Steps*, holding each hand placement for 2 to 5 minutes. Take a half an hour, 45 minutes to an hour and immerse yourself in your palpable relationship with Source, Creative Intelligence energy. Remember to relax your shoulders, arms, hands and fingers and exhale. Exhaling makes room for natural breathing without effort.

Make time for yourself first thing in the morning before you get out of bed or at night before you go to sleep, or sitting at your desk with your elbows on your desk, or riding the bus or train to work. You will find your own ways to enjoy this extraordinary healing art.

Remember, this information is for educational purposes only and not intended to diagnose, prescribe, treat, cure, or replace professional medical care or emergency care of any kind.

The Quick Steps in **bold** may be very helpful for the following specific health projects (listed in italics).

Adrenals Health
  1. **The Central Connection**
  7. **Whole Side Back**
11. Lighten Your Load
13. Love Your Self
23. **Use Your Life Well**
32. Exhaustion Relief

Babies (and Mothers too) Comfort
  1. The Central Connection
15. **Healthy Boundaries**
16. **Nourish and Nurture**
25. **Breathe from Toes to Head**
29. **Protecting Your Organs**
42. **Happy Lungs**

Chemotherapy and Radiation "Ease"
  1. The Central Connection
  7. Whole Side Back
10. Joy, Joy, Joy
15. **Healthy Boundaries**
16. **Nourish and Nurture**
25. Breathe from Toes to Head
29. Protecting Your Organs
32. Exhaustion Relief
44. **The Transformer**

Circulation
  0. **Complete Breath Hug**
  1. The Central Connection
  6. **Whole Side Front**
10. Joy, Joy, Joy
17. Smooth Rhythm and Movement
28. **Uplifts, Brings Vitality, Recharges Heart**
35. **Heart Wholeness**

Elder Health

0. Complete Breath Hug
1. The Central Connection
5. Gives You Wings
8. Dancing Moderator and Emotional Balance
19. Muscle Tone and Weight Balance
23. Use Your Life Well
44. The Transformer
49. Bones Help

Emotional Balancing

0. Complete Breath Hug
1. The Central Connection
4. Big Happy Janitor
8. Dancing Moderator and Emotional Balance
13. Love Your Self
36. Harmonizing Worry
37. Harmonizing Fear
38. Harmonizing Anger
39. Harmonizing Sadness
40. Harmonizing Trying to Do and Be Too Much

Facelift Naturally

4. Big Happy Janitor
11. Lighten Your Load
12. Eyes, Ears, and Balance
14. All Elements Come to Rest Here
15. Healthy Boundaries
26. Compassionate Understanding
27. Decision Making Support
45. Burn Relief

Heart Wholeness

0. Complete Breath Hug
1. The Central Connection

High "De-Anxiety"

29. Protecting Your Organs
30. Take What You Need and Dump the Rest
35. Heart Wholeness
41. Harmonizing Trying to Do and Be Too Much

High "De-Anxiety"

0. Complete Breath Hug
1. The Central Connection
23. Use Your Life Well
24. Waist Up-Waist Down Harmony
34. Calms Nervous System
41. Harmonizing Trying to Do and Be Too Much
47. Personal Analgesic

Hormonal Health

1. The Central Connection
10. Joy, Joy, Joy
28. Uplifts, Brings Vitality, Recharges Heart
29. Protecting Your Organs
30. Take What You Need and Dump the Rest
35. Heart Wholeness

Pain Relief

0. Complete Breath Hug
17. Smooth Rhythm and Movement
41. Magnificent Circulation
44. The Transformer
46. Moving Pains
47. Personal Analgesic

Pre- and Post Surgery "Ease"

0. Complete Breath Hug
1. The Central Connection
16. Nourish and Nurture

25. Breathe from Toes to Head
34. Calms Nervous System
41. Magnificent Circulation

Soldier's Relief
0. Complete Breath Hug
1. The Central Connection
2. Higher Wisdom
8. Dancing Moderator and Emotional Balance
15. Healthy Boundaries
22. Comfortable Wherever You Are
24. Waist Up-Waist Down Harmony (Brain stress)
28. Uplifts, Brings Vitality, Recharges Heart
29. Protecting Your Organs
35. Heart Wholeness
36. Harmonizing Worry
37. Harmonizing Fear
38. Harmonizing Anger
39. Harmonizing Sadness
40. Harmonizing Trying to Do and Be Too Much

Stroke "Free" Zone
22. Comfortable Wherever You Are
24. Waist Up-Waist Down Harmony
25. Breathe from Toes to Head
44. The Transformer

Teenagers' "Comfort"
0. Complete Breath Hug
2. Higher Wisdom
3. The Great Movement
8. Dancing Moderator and Emotional Balance
15. Healthy Boundaries

23. Use Your Life Well
24. Waist Up-Waist Down Harmony
45. Burn Relief

Thyroid Health
1. The Central Connection
5. Gives You Wings
11. Lighten your Load
12. Eyes, Ears and Balance
13. Love Your Self
18. Helps Everything
22. Comfortable Wherever You Are

Vitality
5. Gives You Wings
16. Nourish and Nurture
23. Use Your Life Well
28. Uplifts, Brings Vitality, Recharges Heart
32. Exhaustion Relief

Weight Loss "Ease"
1. The Central Connection
6. Whole Side Front
7. Whole Side Back
9. Completing and Beginning
13. Love Your Self
15. Healthy Boundaries
16. Nourish and Nurture
18. Helps Everything
19. Muscle Tone and Weight Balance
24. Waist Up –Waist Down Balance
28. Uplifts, Brings Vitality, Recharges Heart

There you have it!

Starting from zero and going through 49 *Healing Touch Quick Steps*, you now have "50 ways to love yourself" or maybe more precisely, "50 ways to receive love from the Universe."

In 1994 and for a couple of years after that I was blessed to receive regular *Jin Shin Jyutsu* healing sessions from Mary Burmeister, the woman who brought *Jin Shin Jyutsu* to the United States. (Mary passed away in January, 2008.)

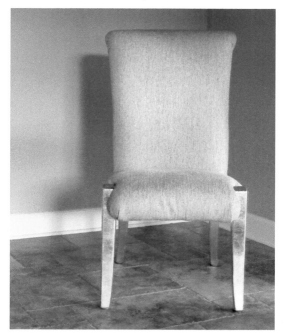

I was pretty sick when I first came to see Mary. I would hear her say out loud, *"Please take care for her, God."* Then she would continue in silence, listening to my body's pulses respond. Soon after her request of God to help me, I'd hear her say out loud, *"Thank you, God."* Often I would hear her simply say, *"Thank you, God,"* as if she'd already asked in silence for God to again please take care of me, and she'd heard God's response in my pulses almost instantly even when I was so sick. Mary Burmeister had a very close working relationship with God.

When you do your *Healing Touch Quick Steps* self-help, consider making the name of the *Healing Touch Quick Step* you are applying an "active prayer." For example, *"Please take care of me [God, or whatever that is for you] with **Healthy Boundaries**. Thank you [God or whatever that is for you]."* Or if you do not want to say "please" and you'd rather set it up as an intention, you can say, *"I am choosing wholeness now for my digestive system with this **Healthy Boundaries** Quick Step."* Feel free to enjoy and be creative with this healing art. I like the idea of "actively praying" and choosing wholeness when I am giving myself these *Healing Touch Quick Steps.*

With the application of *Healing Touch Quick Steps*, you may have become aware of a presence, a state of being in

Oneness, wholeness, perfect health, instant healing, some graceful response, a Source that is pulsing through your whole being, maybe even as an "*experience of supreme unconditional love*" that *Eat, Pray, Love* author Elizabeth Gilbert describes as her definition for the word God.

Instant healing is a state of being that IS a cure for what ails you. Instant healing is a new wave of understanding that you and Source are one, and a part of you exists beyond physical disease.

With the current science expanding and proving that in a hundredth of a second based on what you think, feel and say you can shift your body-mind chemistry, and when each person chooses to deepen her own personal interactions with Source, who knows, maybe humans are actually evolving into a realm of wholeness in which we can choose to "flip a switch" to the perfect health part of us to replace a "dis-eased" part of the body?

All goodness, some even say magic or miracles, is possible when you are in a committed relationship with Source.

What I know for sure is that through *Healing Touch Quick Steps* you now have know-how to connect with universal energy, the unified field, holistic system of Big Picture life force that is bigger than any worldly disturbance. Your "inner" and your "outer" are connected.

You can return to neutral often.
Choose wholeness regularly.
Look for your harmony everyday.
BE the harmony!

Remember now you are focusing on what strengthens you. When you come from a place of kindness for yourself, your compassionate body awareness engages you in the present moment. And, that's a good thing.

As a free gift, you may go to my website: **www.healingtouchquicksteps.com** and download the audio CD called "*Secrets to Stress Relief.*" Enjoy!

Many blessings I send to you for your health and wholeness.

–Barbara J. Semple

66 *What I call the 'inner body' isn't really the body anymore but life energy, the bridge between form and formless.*

Make it a habit to feel the inner body as often as you can. When you are in touch with the inner body, you are not identified with your body anymore, nor are you identified with your mind... **99**

–Eckhart Tolle, *A New Earth – Awakening Your Life's Purpose*

Bibliography

Bainbridge Cohen, Bonnie. 1993. *Sensing, Feeling and Action – The Experiential Anatomy of Body-Mind Centering*. Northampton, Contact Editions.

Braden, Gregg. 2005. *The God Code – The Secret of Our Past, the Promise of Our Future*. Hay House.

Burmeister, Alice. 1997. *The Touch of Healing – Energizing Body, Mind, and Spirit with the Art of Jin Shin Jyutsu®*. New York, Toronto, London, Sydney, Auckland, Bantam Books..

Burmeister, Mary. 1985, 1994. *Introducing Jin Shin Jyutsu, Book 1*. Scottsdale, JSJ Distributors.

—————. 1981. *Introducing Jin Shin Jyutsu, Book 2*. Scottsdale, JSJ Distributors.

—————. 1985. *Introducing Jin Shin Jyutsu, Book 3*. Scottsdale, JSJ Distributors.

—————. 1971-1997. *Text II-Physio-Philosophy*. Scottsdale, Jin Shin Jyutsu, Inc.

—————. 1997. *What Mary Says*. Scottsdale, JSJ, Inc.

CanWest News Service. September 30, 2005. Article: *Job stress takes its toll on the Brain*.

Chopra, Deepak, M.D. 1991-2000. *Perfect Health – The Complete Mind Body Guide*. New York, Three Rivers Press.

—————. 2006. *Power, Freedom and Grace: Living from the Source of Lasting Happiness*. San Rafael, Amber-Allen Publishing, Inc.

Connelly, Dianne M., Ph.D., M.Ac. 1993, 1986. *All Sickness is Homesickness*. Columbia, Traditional Acupuncture Institute.

—————. 1989, 1979. *Traditional Acupuncture: The Law of the Five Elements*. Columbia, Traditional Acupuncture Institute.

De Rodriguez, Gary. 2008. *From my notes from his seminar* in May, 2008. New Mexico, Life Design International. www.garyderodriguez.com

Emoto, Masaru. 2004. *The Hidden Messages in Water*. Hillsboro, Beyond Words Publishing.

Field, Melinda and Phillips, Lani. 2004. Wisdom of the Crone Cards. Mount Shasta, www.wisdomofthecrone.com.

Gach, Michael Reed. 1989. *Arthritis Relief at Your Fingertips – The Complete Guide to Easing Aches and Pains Without Drugs*. New York, Warner Books.

Hammer, Leon, M.D. 1990. *Dragon Rises, Red Bird Flies – Psychology, Energy & Chinese Medicine*. New York, Station Hill Press.

HERBS AND MEDICINAL PLANTS KNOWLEDGE CARDSTM. No date given. The Academy of Natural Sciences, Philadelphia, PA.

Iglehart Austen, Hallie. 1991, 1990. *The Heart of the Goddess – Art, Myth and Meditations of the World's Sacred Feminine*. Berkeley, Wingbow Press.

Jiyu-Kennett, Roshi and MacPhillamy, Rev. Daizui. 1979. *The Book of Life*. Mt. Shasta, Shasta Abbey Press.

Kaptchuk, Ted J., O.M.D. 1983. *The Web Has No Weaver – Understanding Chinese Medicine*. New York, Congdon & Weed, Inc.

Lipton, Bruce H., Ph.D. 2005. *The Biology of Belief – Unleashing the Power of Consciousness, Matter, and Miracles*. Santa Rosa, Mountain of Love/Elite Books.

Matsumoto, Kiiko, and Birch, Stephen. 1983. *Five Elements and Ten Stems – Nan Ching Theory*, Diagnostics and Practice. Brookline, Paradigm Publications.

McTaggart, Lynne. 2008. *Living the Field: Earth Energies Report*.

—————. 2008. *Living the Field Handout: The Science of the Field*.

—————. 2007. *The Intention Experiment: Using Your Thoughts to Change Your Life and the World*. New York, Free Press, Simon & Schuster.

Moss, Nan and Corbin, David. 2008. *Weather Shamanism: Harmonizing Our Connection with the Elements*. Rochester, Vermont. Bear & Company.

Motz, Julie. 1998. *Hands of Life: Using Your Body's Own Energy Medicine for Healing, Recovery, and Transformation*. New York, Bantam Books.

Nunn, John F. 1996. *Ancient Egyptian Medicine*. Red River Books, University of Oklahoma Press: Norman.

Oz, Mehmet C., M.D. with Ron Arias and Lisa Oz. 1998. *Healing from the Heart: A Leading Surgeon Reveals How Unconventional Wisdom Unleashes the Power of Modern Medicine*. New York, Penguin Group.

Pinkola-Estes, PhD, Clarissa. 1992. *Women Who Run With the Wolves: Myths and Stories of the Wild Woman Archetype*. New York, Ballantine.

Ristad, Eloise. 1982. *A Soprano on Her Head: Right-side up reflections on life and other performances*. Moab, Real People Press.

Saunders, E.Dale. 1985, 1960. *Mudra – A Study of Symbolic Gestures in Japanese Buddhist Sculpture*. Princeton, Princeton University Press.

Serizawa, Katsusuke, M.D. 1976. *TSUBO – Vital Points for Oriental Therapy*. Tokyo, Japan Publications, Inc.

Shames, Richard, M.D. and Shames, Karilee, Ph.D, RN. 2005. *Feeling Fat, Fuzzy, and Frazzled? – A 3 Step Program to Beat Hormone Havoc, Restore Thyroid, Adrenal, and Reproductive Balance, Feel Better Fast*. New York, Hudson Street Press, Penguin Group.

Supreme Grand Lodge of the Ancient & Mystical Order Rosæ Crucis. *Mystic Wisdom: Insiration for the Soul*. 2008. San Jose, AMORC, Inc.

Taylor, Jill Bolte, PhD. 2006. *My Stroke of Insight: A Brain Scientist's Personal Journey*. New York, Viking, Penguin Group.

Thie, John F., D.C. 1987, 1977. *Touch For Health*. Pasadena, T.H. Enterprises, Publishers.

Tolle, Eckhart. 2005. *A New Earth: Awakening Your Life's Purpose*. New York. Dutton, Penguin Group.

Viegas, Jennifer. 2006, July. "Hands shown to emit light." *Discovery News*.

Vieth, Ilza. 1972, 1966, 1949. *The Yellow Emperor's Classic of Internal Medicine*. Berkeley, Los Angeles, London, University of California Press.

Multi-Media Home Study Program from Barbara J. Semple. . .

Healing Touch Quick Steps HOME GUIDE – 42 Powerful Things You Can Do Instantly to Bring Your Body into Harmony

"This thing ROCKS! It is immediate, easy to use, and you can do it in the flow of life, whatever is going on. This is so precious." - Louise Deerfield, Entrepreneur

Your Healing Touch Quick Steps HOME GUIDE program includes all of this:

1. Top 10 Healing Touch Quick Steps DVD: 55 minutes with soothing music, beautiful Nature visuals and healthy, happy models showing you where to place your hands on your body instantly.
2. Slide show of 42 Healing Touch Quick Steps with complete audio commentaries.
3. 71 page eBook including full color pictures, descriptions and an extensive interactive INDEX for over 1,000 symptoms that may be addressed with the Quick Steps.
4. TRAVELLER'S Aid Audio CD with 8 specific Quick Steps to encourage circulation, relaxation and vitality while traveling, plus picture reference card.
5. SOLDIER'S Relief Audio CD with 9 Quick Steps self-help for soldiers, nurses, emergency room doctors, crew chiefs, people who work at night, police and highway patrol officers, fire department personnel, prison guards, and even prisoners – anyone who deals with other people's pain and chaos everyday, plus picture reference card.
6. EMOTIONAL Balancing Audio CD with 9 Quick Steps for young and old to engage emotional health and well being, plus picture reference card.
7. Secrets to Stress Relief Audio CD: An Interview with Self-Healing Advocate Barbara J. Semple gives

background and historical information about healing with Nature.

8. PRE- and POST Surgery Picture Reference Card with 7 Healing Touch Quick Steps. The simpler, the better.
9. COLD FLU Relief Picture Reference Card with 7 Healing Touch Quick Steps for easing symptoms.
10. Three (3) Quick, Quicker and Quickest Reference Cards for choosing particular symptomatic instant access plus a Getting Started Guide.

Autobiographical Journey. . .

Soul Aerobics® - Conscious Movement of a Soul into Wholeness

by Barbara J. Semple

Soul Aerobics - Conscious Movement of a Soul into Wholeness is the story of one woman's healing journey consciously choosing to align her little self, ego-personality, with her soul.

With a natural wisdom of transformative healing, Barbara reminds us that wholeness or holiness is our constant state of being even when we are sick. A person need not have a physical ailment to gain inspiration and liberation from this easy-to-read triumphant story.

"Liberally sprinkled with alluring chapter snippets like 'Listening is an Act of Love' and 'Putting It on the Altar to Bleed,' Semple offers convincing instruction to readers in search of a true and timeless 'soul-physical' relationship, or, as the book's subtitle suggests, toward a 'conscious movement of a soul to wholeness.' Soul Aerobics is a gentle and fascinating account of Semple's personal discoveries and journey toward a loving heart, and readers who jump aboard for a ride indeed may find themselves headed for that very same destination as

well. *A lovely book to trust and enjoy."*
thebooxreview.com, July 2002

"Soul Aerobics takes readers straight to the heart of their own authentic power. Barbara's writing is deeply personal, at times lyrical, always uplifting and filled with compassion. I am both moved and educated in the process. This is a superb account of hope, healing and transformation. The great value of this book is that it is written by a woman who has faced extraordinary challenges and lived to enjoy greater strength, wisdom and love in the process. It's a roadmap for the healing journey by an author who knows the path well."
Hal Zina Bennett, author of *Write From the Heart* and *Spirit Animals and the Wheel of Life*

Life-Saving First Creation from Barbara...

Personal Power Cards - Flashcards for Emotional Wellness are available online at www.healingtouchquicksteps.com/products.html.

By Barbara J. Semple

The perfect gift for anyone who needs a little positive self-talk. Barbara says the first 10 cards of this deck are what kept her connected to her soul through her near-death experience in 1988.

Barbara Semple's first published project called *Personal Power Cards - Flashcards for Emotional Wellness*, are available directly online from Compassionate Healing Instruction LLC, or through New Leaf Distributors if you are a bookseller; from your bookstore as a special order, as well as available at amazon.com.

Personal Power Cards include 55 full-color cards the size

and lamination of regular playing cards, a 80 page booklet and a red cotton carrying pouch. *Personal Power Cards* are words the soul might say to you giving its higher perspective of thoughts and feelings. They remind you of the goodness of you, especially when you are in pain or "dis-ease." Here is help you can hold in your hand to engage the multi-sensory brain and mind.

"When I used these cards, I felt more calm and centered, which fits with [Semple]'s suggestion that the cards can also be used to relieve momentary stress. This is a powerful deck to offer to people who want to retrain their responses to life, and one of the most useful recovery tools I have seen."
New Age Retailer Review

"Personal Power Cards are the greatest advance in diagnosis by light since the Lüscher Color Test. In the twenty years I have been using color and mind imagery with patients, I have never seen any approach have such a great benefit on self-discipline and self-esteem. Using the system's five categories of wellness, one may get a stronger handle on overall health than by any other single technique. Personal Power Cards can make well-being a new habit for many, many people."
Richard Shames, M.D., family practitioner and author of *Healing With Mind Power and Thyroid Power*

"Personal Power Cards symbolically reinforce the power of intention. A valuable tool for affirming personal, professional and spiritual goals."
Angeles Arrien, author of *Signs of Life* and the *Handbook of Tarot*

In 1988 at age 34, after a near-death experience, 5 days in intensive care, and a serious strep infection, Barbara J. Semple was diagnosed with severe rheumatoid arthritis. Back then there was little known about how to help a person dealing with rheumatoid arthritis. From this challenging period of deep soul searching, Barbara came forth choosing life, love and joy. And, she says a funny thing happened after losing everything in the prime of her life while being forced by her body to pay 100% attention to it. "*The more present I was with my body's needs and care, the more I felt a sense of wholeness and spirituality. My body has taught me a lot about living with ease and grace*," says Barbara.

Today, Barbara is an integrative healing arts practitioner specializing in the art of *Jin Shin Jyutsu*®, teacher of energy self-help, and a *Certified Laughter Yoga*® *Leader*. She is author of a number of books including **Soul Aerobics® - Conscious Movement of a Soul Into Wholeness.** Her first published work, **Personal Power Cards – Flash Cards for Emotional Wellness** set a tone for easy-to-use self-help tools long before any other card sets were available on the market. New Age Retailer called Barbara's **Personal Power Cards** "*one of the most useful recovery tools ever seen.*" Barbara is also author of the multi-media home study program called **Healing Touch Quick Steps HOME GUIDE – 42 Powerful Things You Can Do Instantly to Bring Your Body into Harmony.**

Barbara's website is:
www.healingtouchquicksteps.com.

To order additional copies of this book, contact:
Xlibris Corporation
1-888-795-4274
www.Xlibris.com
Orders@Xlibris.com

Lightning Source UK Ltd.
Milton Keynes UK
UKHW051429260619
345043UK00003B/12/P